Investing in Communities Achieves Results

DIRECTIONS IN DEVELOPMENT
Human Development

Investing in Communities Achieves Results

Findings from an Evaluation of Community Responses to HIV and AIDS

Rosalía Rodriguez-García, René Bonnel, David Wilson, and N'Della N'Jie

THE WORLD BANK
Washington, D.C.

Contents

Boxes

Figures

Tables

Acknowledgments

This synthesis paper was prepared under the leadership of Rosalía Rodriguez-García, M.Sc., Ph.D., Team Leader, Evaluation of the Community Response to HIV and AIDS, World Bank. The report is based on the totality of country and desk studies that were produced as part of the evaluation of the community response to HIV and AIDS conducted in partnership with the United Kingdom's Department for International Development (DfID) and the UK Consortium on AIDS and International Development (UK Consortium).

The overall evaluation exercise was led by Rosalía Rodriguez-García with René Bonnel and N'Della N'Jie at the World Bank; Louise Robinson, Silke Seco-Grutz, Anna Seymour, and Andrea Cook from DfID; and Ben Simms from the UK Consortium. The country evaluations were designed and implemented with national researchers, national AIDS authorities, World Bank and DfID country teams, partners, and civil society representatives.

World Bank researchers Markus Goldstein, Damien de Walque, Ariana Legovini, and Quentin Wodon contributed to specific studies. The evaluation benefited from the support of David Wilson, Director of the HIV/AIDS Program, and Jody Zall Kusek, AIDS Cluster Leader, Health, Nutrition and Population, World Bank, as well as Nick York, Head of Evaluation, DfID. Thanks are due to Cristian Baeza, Director and Nicole Klingen, Sector Manager of Health Nutrition and Population, and Brian Pascual, Uma Balasubramanian, and Mario Mendez from the Human Development Network, World Bank. Kate Bigmore, Marcelo Bortman, Rafael Cortez, Daniel Cotlear, Montserrat Meiro-Lorenzo, Michael O'Dwyer, Aakanksha Pande, Anne M. Pierre-Louis, Iris Semini, and Quentin Wodon provided very useful early comments. Special thanks to Corinne Low (Columbia University) for her valuable insights and contributions.

Most important, this evaluation is the product of a team effort with researchers from inside and outside of the World Bank. The lead researchers are recognized below (in alphabetical order by last name). More information on study teams and reports can be found in appendix A. A list of peer reviewers of this and other evaluation products is included in appendix B. To all, we express our sincere appreciation.

- *Burkina Faso*: Damien de Walque (World Bank)
- *India:* T. L. Mohan (Karnataka Health Promotion Trust KHPT), Stephen Moses (University of Manitoba), and Tisha Wheeler (The Bill and Melinda Gates Foundation)
- *Kenya*: Marcus Goldstein (World Bank), Jakub Kakietek (ICF Macro), Paul Kizito (National Coordinating Agency for Population and Development), Bruce Larson (Boston University), Corinne Low (Columbia University), Brigitte Manteuffel (ICF Macro), and Alloys Orago (National AIDS Control Council)
- *Lesotho*: Damien de Walque (World Bank)
- *Nigeria*: Sani Ali Gar and Inuwa Jalingo (National Population Commission), Jakub Kakietek and Brigitte Manteuffel (ICF Macro), and Kayode Ogungbemi (National Agency for the Control of AIDS)
- *Senegal*: Jean-Louis Arcand (The Graduate Institute, Geneva) and Ariana Legovini (World Bank)
- *South Africa*: Damien de Walque (World Bank)
- *Zimbabwe*: Cathy Campbell (London School of Economics and Political Science), Simon Gregson (Imperial College, London, and Biomedical Research and Training Institute), Tapuwa Magure (National AIDS Council), Constance Nyamukapa (Imperial College, London, and Biomedical Research and Training Institute), and Lorraine Sherr (University College, London)

Our thanks also go to the UK Consortium on AIDS and International Development and its network for their tireless support and contributions to this evaluation, particularly to the Board of Directors: Dieneke ter Huurne, International Planned Parenthood Foundation; Mike Podmore, International HIV/AIDS Alliance; Alan Smith, Interact Worldwide; Nikki Jeffery, Target Tuberculosis; Nina O'Farrell, Christian Aid; and Dermott McDonald, Mildmay International. Our appreciation goes to the International AIDS Alliance for supporting funding flows analysis and value-for-money thinking.

We would also like to recognize the support of partners who accompanied the evaluation process and provided sound advice. These include: UNAIDS Secretariat, USAID, The Bill and Melinda Gates Foundation, The Global Fund, the U.S. President's Emergency Plan for AIDS Relief (PEPFAR), the United Nations Children's Fund (UNICEF), and other UNAIDS cosponsoring agencies.

The opinions expressed in this report are those of the authors, who are responsible for interpretations and any omissions. The findings, interpretations, and conclusions expressed in this volume do not necessarily reflect the views of the Executive Directors of the World Bank or the governments they represent.

This work has been partially funded by UKaid, the UK Department for International Development; however, the views expressed do not necessarily reflect the department's official policies.

Abbreviations

AIDS	Acquired immune deficiency syndrome
AMPATH	Academic Model Providing Access to Healthcare
ART	Antiretroviral therapy
ARV	Antiretroviral
BCC	Behavioral change communication
BTS	Behavioral Tracking Survey
CBO	Community-based organization
CCT	Conditional cash transfers
CDD	Community-driven development
CSO	Civil society organization
DfID	Department for International Development (UK)
DHS	Demographic and Health Survey
EIC	Education, information, and communication
FBO	Faith-based organization
FEATS	Effective AIDS Treatment and Support in the Free State
FSW	Female sex worker
HIV	Human immunodeficiency virus
HBC	Home-based care
HBCT	Home-based counseling and testing
HCT	HIV counseling and testing
HLFPPT	Hindustan Latex Family Planning Promotion Trust
IBBA	Integrated Behavioral and Biological Assessment
IDU	Injecting drug user
IEC	Information and education campaign
IEG	Independent evaluation group (World Bank)
KHPT	Karnataka Health Promotion Trust (India)
KSAPS	Karnataka State AIDS Prevention Society
LDHS	Lesotho Demographic and Health Survey

MAP	Multi-Country HIV/AIDS Program
MSM	Men who have sex with men
MSM/Ts	Men who have sex with men and transgender individuals
NAC	National AIDS Commissions
NACA	National Agency for the Control of AIDS
NASA	National AIDS Spending Assessment
NGO	Nongovernmental organization
OED	Operations Evaluation Department (World Bank)
OVC	Orphans and vulnerable children
PEPFAR	President's Emergency Plan for AIDS Relief (U.S.)
PLWHA	People living with HIV and AIDS
PMTCT	Prevention of mother-to-child transmission
PSM	Propensity score matching
QUIBB	Questionnaire on Basic Welfare Indicators
RCT	Randomized control trial
STI	Sexually transmitted infection
SW	Sex worker
UCT	Unconditional cash transfers
UK Consortium	UK Consortium on AIDS and International Development
UNAIDS	Joint United Nations Programme on HIV/AIDS
UNGASS	United Nations General Assembly Special Session on HIV/AIDS
WHO	World Health Organization

Note: All dollar amounts are U.S. dollars unless otherwise stated.

Overview

Abstract

The Overview summarizes the evaluation of community responses (15 studies, including 11 evaluations carried out in 8 countries). It presents the evaluation questions, the methodology, the key results achieved by community responses along the continuum of prevention, treatment, care and support, and the resulting policy and programmatic implications.

Introduction

Before the scale-up of the international response to the AIDS pandemic, community responses in developing countries played a crucial role in providing services and care for those affected. This study is the first comprehensive, mixed-method evaluation of the impact of that response. The evaluation finds that community response can be effective at increasing knowledge of HIV, promoting social empowerment, increasing access to and use of HIV services, and even decreasing HIV incidence, all through the effective mobilization of limited resources. By effectively engaging with this powerful community structure, future HIV and AIDS programs can ensure that communities continue to contribute to the global response to HIV and AIDS.

Background

Since the beginning of the Human Immunodeficiency Virus and the Acquired Immune Deficiency Syndrome (HIV and AIDS) epidemic, communities have played an important role in addressing the HIV and AIDS challenge, often working in tandem with governments. Communities have been instrumental in developing innovative approaches to service uptake and delivery and in accessing and empowering marginalized populations affected by the epidemic. Community-based organizations (CBOs) have long been at the forefront of the global movement to address the epidemic. The first organizational responses came, almost universally, from affected individuals, their families, and community groups—the community response.[1] Civil society organizations (CSOs), which include nongovernmental organizations (NGOs) and CBOs, now represent a complex, international network working along the entire continuum of prevention, care, treatment, and support.

Simultaneously in the first decade of the twenty-first century, the demand for development effectiveness swept through the international community, raising expectations about achieving measurable and tangible results on the ground, and demonstrating the impact of these results. The importance of rigorous evaluation efforts that would be closely linked to national policy-making, involve stakeholders, increase the knowledge base, and improve operations became part of the global dialogue. Yet many of the activities of civil society were not always the focus of rigorous evaluations, which often concentrated on measuring project or specific intervention impacts. The broad nature of community organization and action clashes with the struc-tured methodology of impact evaluations. Thus, the effects of community-based activities on the communities and population groups they serve, remained largely unmeasured.

Context and Evaluation Questions

Between 2002 and 2008 the AIDS response experienced a rapid, more than six-fold increase in donor disbursements. Then, after several years of flat funding, in 2011 donor governments disbursed US$7.6 billion for the AIDS response in low- and middle-income countries (Kaiser Family Foundation 2012). These disbursements support a global response to an epidemic that has claimed 35 million lives from AIDS-related causes since the disease was first reported 31 years ago; by the end of 2011, about 34.2 million people were living with AIDS (Kaiser Family Foundation and UNAIDS 2012) The international donor community has come to recognize the important role played by nongovernmental actors, especially in developing successful approaches to reach the most-affected, high-risk populations. Thus, from 2003 to 2009, the world's four major HIV and AIDS donors—the United Kingdom's Department for International Development (DfID), the Global Fund to Fight AIDS, Tuberculosis and Malaria (the Global Fund), the U.S. President's Emergency Plan for AIDS Relief (PEPFAR), and the World Bank disbursed about one-third of their AIDS support budget through CSOs, large and small. These organizations have been used by donors and governments to help deliver on their strategies and programs in support of community responses to the HIV epidemic (Kaiser Family Foundation 2011). The Global Fund alone reported that by end of the 2009 reporting cycle, one-third of US$6.8 billion in country expenditures was implemented by CSOs and aca-demia (Global Fund 2011).

Recognizing the need for a better understanding of the impact of community responses, the World Bank and DfID launched the evaluation reported here in 2009. The overarching question of the evaluation was: *What results have investments produced at the community level?* In this context, the evaluation examined the following key questions:

1. How do the flow of funds to communities and the allocation of funding by CBOs contribute to community responses and to the national response to HIV and AIDS?
2. Do community responses result in improved knowledge and behavior?
3. Do community responses result in increased access to and utilization of services?
4. Do community responses result in observable social transformation?[2]
5. Can these factors combine to decrease HIV incidence and improve health outcomes?

Using a variety of methodologies, instruments, and country settings, the portfolio of 15 studies has produced rich and illuminating results helpful to policymakers, researchers, civil society, and evaluators. This document analyzes and synthesizes the findings. The approach and the findings on community-level results aims to be useful and applicable to other sectors and thematic areas.

Audience

The audience for this paper is a broad one, including, among others, national AIDS authorities, bilateral and multilateral donors, community representatives, civil society, researchers, and academicians. Ultimately the evaluation aims to build knowledge about community-based activities and results to better inform donors, governments, civil society, and communities and help guide their decisions about resource allocations and program structuring.

Methodology

This evaluation has collected substantial and wide-ranging field data. Thus, the analysis of findings is based on current primary data—quantitative, qualitative, and financial. In some instances, primary data were complemented by new analyses of secondary data. Given the vast range and variety of community responses, this evaluation applied a mixed-method, multicountry, portfolio approach implemented by multidisciplinary teams of researchers. The evaluation exercise comprised a total of 17 studies, which included country-specific evaluations in Burkina Faso, India, Kenya, Lesotho, Nigeria, Senegal, South Africa, and Zimbabwe. These countries were selected for their diversity of epidemic status[3] (generalized versus concentrated), HIV prevalence, and geographic location.

The methodology varied across countries as a function of the specific research questions to be studied and the respective context. Some studies used an experimental design (e.g., randomized control trial—RCT) with individual, household, or community randomization. Some studies were quasi-experimental, using repeated cross-sectional surveys and matching methods to establish comparison groups. The experimental and quasi-experimental studies used robust methods for establishing a "counterfactual" meaning: What would have happened to a similar group of people in the absence of community intervention? Other studies used descriptive and analytical methods. Most country studies also collected a range of qualitative (social transformation) and financial (flow of funds) data. Desk studies reviewed existing documentation as well as new survey data to inform and complement the country evaluations. By using several methods, the limitations of any particular method were mitigated. A process of expert review and consultation was instrumental in managing the limitations presented by the overall portfolio approach.

This evaluation defines *community* as a shared *cultural identity* (members belong to a group that shares common characteristics or interests) or as a *geographic place* (a group in a physical location or an administrative entity). *Community response* is defined as the combination of actions and steps taken by communities, including the provision of goods and services, to prevent and/or address a problem and to bring about social change. Community responses can be characterized in six main categories: (a) types of implementing organizations and structures; (b) types of implemented activities or services and beneficiaries; (c) actors involved in and driving the response; (d) contextual factors influencing responses; (e) the extent of community involvement in the response; and (f) the extent of involvement of wider partnerships and collaborative efforts (Rodriguez-García et al. 2011). These classifications were applied by the studies to define different types or aspects of community responses.

A consultative peer review process was embedded in the evaluation at the global, national, and local levels with experts, academics, partner organizations, civil society groups, and other stakeholders. As noted, this consultative process helped ensure the rigor of the evaluation. Civil society consultations were facilitated by a purposeful partnership with the UK Consortium on AIDS and International Development.[4]

Findings

The evaluation found evidence (varying from causal to associative to suggestive) that, depending on the country context and service delivery mechanisms, the response of communities can achieve the following:

Help Mobilize Substantial Local Resources

As mentioned before, during 2003–2009 international funding for civil society was significant, reaching more than US$690 million per year (Bonnel et al. 2011). By the end of their 2009 reporting cycle, The Global Fund reports that one third of US$6.8 billion in country expenditures was implemented by CSOs and academia (Global Fund 2011). Despite these levels of funding, the funds reaching CBOs remains small: on average US$15,000 per year per CBO in

Kenya, and US$17,000 per year per CBO in Nigeria (Kenya Evaluation Report 2011; Nigeria Evaluation Report 2011).[5]

- The resources mobilized by national funding channels, including governments, foundations, charities and self-fundraising activities, have become crucial sources of funding for CBOs (figure O.1).
- Volunteers are a crucial resource for CBOs. Unpaid volunteers alone add an estimated 56 percent, on average, to CBO budgets in Kenya, Nigeria, and Zimbabwe (table O.1).

Improve Knowledge and Behavior

- Increased HIV knowledge (Kenya) (figure O.2)
- Increased use of condoms (Kenya, India, Zimbabwe)
- Reduced number of sex partners (Zimbabwe)
- Increased testing by the partners of HIV-positive individuals (Senegal)

A key characteristic of successful knowledge-building programs is the intensity of community mobilization. Participation in community groups and frequent discussion of HIV and AIDS-related issues are two important characteristics of effective community activities (Zimbabwe Evaluation Report 2011a, 2011b, 2012). These activities empower groups at high risk of infection, such as female sex workers (FSWs) and men who have sex with men (MSM). This, in turn, can lead to behavioral changes such as condom use in India ($p < .05$) (India Evaluation Report 2012a, 2012b). However, the protective effects of group membership are not automatically guaranteed (Zimbabwe Evaluation Report 2011a). The groups need to be purposeful. The effects worked with women but not with men.

It should be noted, however, that the effects of community responses on knowledge and behaviors are weaker in Burkina Faso and Nigeria. One possible explanation is that knowledge was already high in Nigeria and other factors (such as mass media) provided a more important source of information. In Burkina Faso, prevention activities had an effect on knowledge that varied by gender.

Increase the Use of Services

- Prevention, treatment, care, and support, primarily in rural areas[6] (Nigeria, figure O.3)
- HIV counseling and testing (HCT) (Senegal, Zimbabwe)
- Home-based counseling and testing (HBCT) (Kenya, figure O.4)
- Prevention of mother-to-child transmission (PMTCT) (Zimbabwe)
- Anti-retroviral therapy (ART) by improving timeliness of clinic and hospital visits (South Africa)
- Sexually transmitted infections (STIs) for FSW (India)

Figure O.1 Funding Channels Mobilized by CBOs

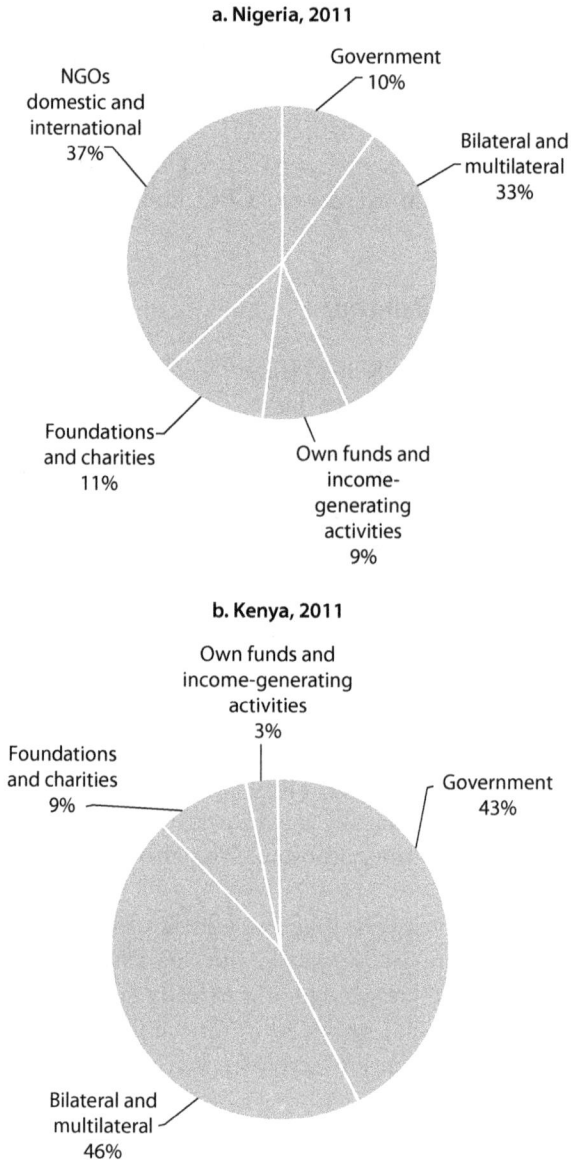

a. Nigeria, 2011

NGOs domestic and international 37%

Government 10%

Bilateral and multilateral 33%

Foundations and charities 11%

Own funds and income-generating activities 9%

b. Kenya, 2011

Own funds and income-generating activities 3%

Foundations and charities 9%

Government 43%

Bilateral and multilateral 46%

Sources: Kenya Evaluation Report 2011; Nigeria Evaluation Report 2011.
Note: CBO = community-based organization; NGO = nongovernmental organization.

Table O.1 Value of Unpaid Volunteers as Percentage of CBO/NGO Budgets

	Kenya	*Nigeria*	*Zimbabwe*
Number of volunteers per CBO/NGO	21	58	196
Value of unpaid volunteers' free labor as percentage of CBO/NGO budgets	40%	48%	69%

Source: Katietek 2012.
Note: CBO = community-based organization; NGO = nongovernmental organization.

Figure O.2 CBO Engagement and HIV Knowledge Improvements in Kenya (Odds of Increase), 2011

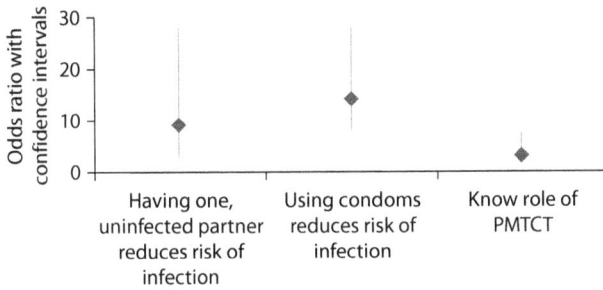

Source: Kenya Evaluation Report 2011.
Note: Diamond = adjusted odds ratio, Line = 95 percent confidence interval, CBO = community-based organization, PMTCT = prevention of mother-to-child transmission.

Figure O.3 CBO Density and Services Use in Rural Areas of Nigeria (Odds of Utilization), 2011

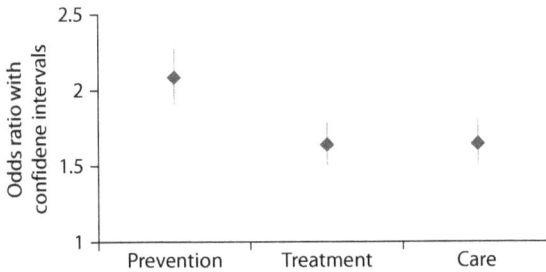

Source: Nigeria Evaluation Report 2011.
Note: Diamond = odds ratio, Line = 95 percent confidence ratio. CBO = community-based organization.

Figure O.4 Percentage of Individuals Who Have Ever Had an HIV Test Due to HBCT

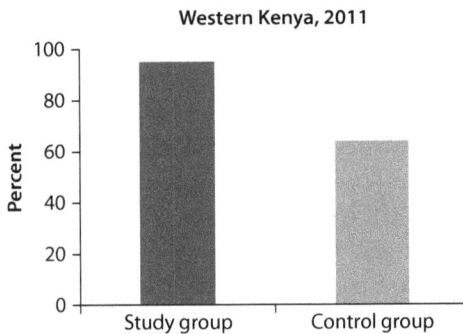

Source: Kenya HBCT Evaluation Report 2012.
Note: HBCT = home-based counseling and testing.

These results indicate that community responses can increase the demand for health services in the context of generalized and concentrated HIV epidemics among groups at high risk of infection. Dedicated support from community members and caregivers, such as peer mentoring, is effective—more so than with "less-personalized" approaches. However, the issue of stigma remains a major hurdle to increasing the use of prevention, treatment, and care in general. Likewise, a socially or legally repressive environment stifles access to health services by the most at-risk populations, such as MSM and transgender individuals (MSM/T) in particular (India Evaluation Report 2012b). Focused research is needed on the area of stigma.

Also of note is the case of access to services in Nigeria. The effects of CBO engagement were most noticeable in rural areas: an increase of one in the number of CBOs per 100,000 people was associated with a twofold increase in the odds that a respondent would report using prevention services, and a 64 percent increase in the odds of reporting treatment access. This finding was stronger in rural communities, where 44 percent were aware of any service, 48 percent of prevention services, and 31 percent of treatment services as compared to 19, 26, and 16 percent for the same categories in urban communities (Nigeria Evaluation Report 2011).

Affect Outcomes of Social Processes

- In India, the evaluation found a strong association between empowerment of FSWs and MSM/T and social change. Being a member of a sex worker community group was associated with access to social entitlements ($p < .05$), reduced violence ($p < .001$), and reduced police coercion ($p < .001$) (India Evaluation Report 2011, 2012b).
- Among Zimbabwe's general population, the community response led to significant changes in sexual risk perception and a reduction in stigmatizing attitudes toward people living with HIV and AIDS—women at 2.5 versus an original 5 percent (aOR = 0.6, CI: 0.3–1.0) and men at 3.5 versus 9 percent (aOR = 0.4, CI: 01–0.9) (Zimbabwe Evaluation Report 2011b).
- Evidence was inconclusive concerning gender norms and domestic violence and abuse. There was mixed evidence concerning stigma (Burkina Faso Evaluation Report 2011; Kenya Evaluation Report 2011; Lesotho Evaluation Report 2011; Nigeria Evaluation Report 2011).

These outcomes demonstrate that community responses can foster social changes among those most affected by the HIV epidemic. However, the effects of community-based activities are gender sensitive, suggesting the need to implement programs that are appropriate to reach heterosexual men, heterosexual women, MSM, and/or FSWs (Zimbabwe Evaluation Report 2011a, 2011b, 2012). Finally, governmental policies can make a great difference, whether they are directed toward commercial sex work, MSM, or domestic abuse. For instance, in Kenya community groups were able to effect change by helping enforce a national policy against domestic abuse. Without such a policy, community action could not have been possible or effective.

Impact HIV Incidence and Other Health Outcomes

- Strong associative evidence was found in Zimbabwe that participation in a community group was associated with reduced HIV incidence for women (aIRR = 0.64, CI: 0.43–0.94) during the period 1998–2003 (Zimbabwe Evaluation Report 2011b; see figure S5). In the following period (2003–2008), the decline in HIV incidence may have slowed, credited mostly to changes in behaviors (Halperin et al. 2011).
- An analysis of data from Karnataka State, India (2005 and 2009), indicates that, compared to nonmembership, community group membership was associated with lower prevalence of STIs, such as chlamydia and gonorrhea (aOR = 0.95, $p < .001$) and active syphilis (aOR = 0.98, $p < .05$) among FSWs (India Evaluation Report 2011).

Therefore, we conclude there is evidence that community group membership can affect real health outcomes. However, it appears that the type of group matters; results vary by gender (the result of reduced HIV incidence in Zimbabwe was only present for women), with decreased HIV incidence only among women); and the stage of the HIV epidemic may impact the size of the effect.

Figure O.5 Community Group Participation and HIV Incidence among Women in Zimbabwe, (1998–2003)

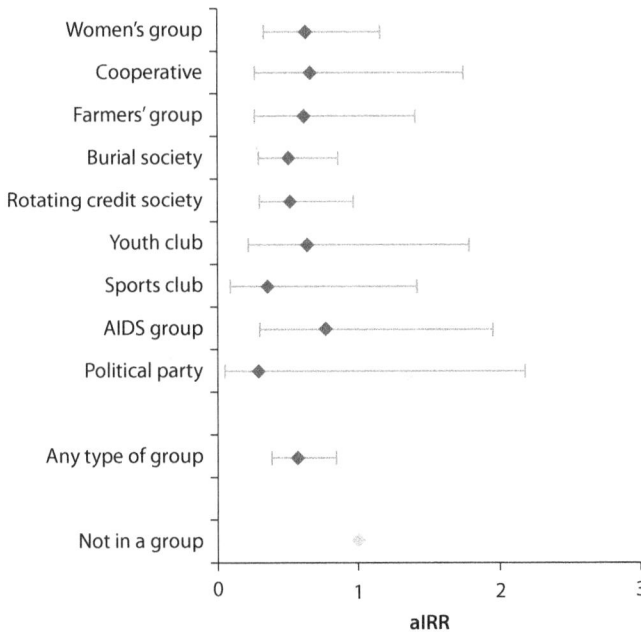

Source: Gregson et al. 2011. Reprinted with permission from the Population Council.
Note: Diamonds = age-adjusted incidence rate ratio (aIRR) and 95 percent confidence interval for HIV infection for individuals in community groups at baseline compared to those not in a group, by form of community group.

Discussion

Table O.2 highlights some of the key findings of the evaluation. It outlines thematic areas and countries where evidence of effects was found, as well as the strength of the evidence. The strongest degree of evidence is provided by experimental studies (RCT) that yield causal evidence of impact. Quasi-experimental and longitudinal studies yield robust evidence with a lower strength. The term "strong associative evidence" is used to characterize these findings. A lower rating (labeled "strong suggestive evidence") is given to quasi-experimental studies that found evidence in only one variation of the indicator, such as in rural areas. Finally, there are cases where the evidence was mixed or inconclusive, such as on gender or stigma issues or where the evaluation did not find a statistically significant effect.

Findings that were not statistically significant might otherwise be programmatically significant. For instance, the National Agency for the Control of AIDS (NACA) in Nigeria pondered why condom use was reportedly low in a country with a high level of HIV knowledge and an NACA national program of condom distribution. While recognizing methodological issues that could be at play, this particular finding generated a useful policy/program dialogue at the country level. Another example is provided by India, where STI incidence among MSM/transgender individuals was not found to be statistically significant. One explanation is that, in this case, real and perceived stigma toward these groups decreased their use of services, and therefore, very few were tested for STIs. Although this evaluation examined community responses to the HIV and AIDS epidemic, the lessons derived through these studies could be applicable to other sectors, especially the health sector. These and other findings are discussed in greater detail in the body of this document.

The following discussion is based primarily on quantitative data supported by qualitative findings. It also incorporates field observations and key informant and expert contributions made during the consultative process of the evaluation at the local, national, and global levels. The discussion of implications aims at generating ideas and dialogue; it is not prescriptive. These implications must be examined in specific contexts if they are to be effective policy arguments. The hope is that these conclusions would be useful to the stakeholders of global, national, and local responses to HIV and AIDS and to those involved in mainstreaming efforts in health and other sectors.

Policy and Programmatic Implications

Program designers need to be savvy about what CBOs and other community actors such as caregivers can realistically achieve. Local response stakeholders can play a critical role by helping communities understand their epidemics and identify priorities for their catchment areas.

A community response cannot become a substitute for a national response. However, communities can help deliver specific results as part of evidence-informed

Table O.2 Highlights of Evidence Concerning the Effects of the Community Response

Activities	Effects	General population	High-risk groups	Strength of evidence
Knowledge				
Information, awareness creation (speaking at public meetings, community theater, and so on)	Increased knowledge about HIV and AIDS	Burkina Faso Kenya Nigeria		Mixed evidence (+/–) Strong associative evidence Not statistically significant
Behaviors				
Promoting use of condoms	Increased condom use	Kenya Nigeria	India	Strong associative evidence Not statistically significant
Peer mentoring for HCT	Increased testing of HIV+ partner	Senegal		Causal evidence
Community group membership	Reduced risk behaviors	Zimbabwe	India	Strong associative evidence
Services				
HIV counseling and testing				
Peer mentoring for HCT	Increased testing and pick up	Senegal		Causal evidence
Group membership (women)	Increased testing	Zimbabwe		Strong associative evidence
Promotion of HCT, mobile HCT	Increased testing	Kenya, Nigeria		Not statistically significant
HBCT	Increased testing	Kenya		Causal evidence
Empowerment of FSWs and MSM	Increased testing		India	Strong associative evidence
Prevention of mother-to-child transmission				
Provision of PMTCT services	Increased use	Zimbabwe		Strong associative evidence
Prevention services and care	Increased use	Nigeria (rural areas)		Strong suggestive evidence
Antiretroviral treatment				
Peer support adherence and nutrition	Increased timeliness of clinic and hospital visits	South Africa		Causal evidence
Care and support				
Awareness of OVC rights Provision of support to OVC	Increased awareness Increased services (rural areas)	Kenya Nigeria		Strong suggestive evidence Strong suggestive evidence
Community group membership	Increased home-based care	Zimbabwe		Strong associative evidence
Mitigation of HIV effect				
Income-generating activities and material support for PLWHA	Increased PLWHA support	Kenya, Nigeria		Not statistically significant

table continues next page

Table O.2 Highlights of Evidence Concerning the Effects of the Community Response (continued)

Activities	Effects	General population	High-risk groups	Strength of evidence
Social change/transformation				
Stigma	Reduced/increased	Burkina Faso, Kenya, Lesotho, Nigeria, Zimbabwe		Mixed evidence
Gender rights, violence	Reduced police violence	Kenya, Nigeria	India	Mixed evidence
Empowerment of groups at high risk of infection	Increased access/ use of social rights		India	Strong associative evidence
AIDS-Health Related Outcomes HIV and AIDS outcomes				
Community group membership	Reduced HIV incidence	Zimbabwe		Strong associative evidence
Empowerment of FSW groups	Lower STI		India	Strong associative evidence
Empowerment of MSM/ Transgender	Lower STI		India	Not statistically significant

Sources: Burkina Faso Evaluation Report 2011; India Evaluation Report 2011, 2012a, 2012b; Kenya Evaluation Report 2011; Kenya HBCT Evaluation Report 2011; Lesotho Evaluation Report 2011; Nigeria Evaluation Report 2011; Senegal Evaluation Report 2010; South Africa Evaluation Report 2011; Zimbabwe Evaluation Report 2011a, 2011b, 2012.
Note: AIDS = acquired immune deficiency syndrome, ART = antiretroviral therapy, FSW = female sex worker, HCT = HIV counseling and testing, HBCT = home-based counseling and testing, HIV = human immunodeficiency virus, MSM = men who have sex with men, OVC = orphans and vulnerable children, PLWHA = people living with HIV and AIDS, PMTCT = prevention of mother-to-child transmission, STI = sexually transmitted infection. (+) = positive effects, (-) = negative effects.

national implementation plans. There needs to be a shift from support of "doing a bit of everything with good intentions" to support for "doing what can be done best with quality." This can take different forms, including:

- *In a context where the epidemic is generalized and reaches high HIV prevalence rates within the general population,* a broad portfolio of community-based activities may be needed to assist in producing the broad social and cultural changes that are required for reversing the course of the epidemic.

- *In contexts where the epidemic combines characteristics of concentrated and generalized epidemics,* community groups and CBOs might have comparative advantages and be able to deliver valuable services. Such services could be focused on (a) specific activities that can complement the national response (e.g., advocacy combined with referrals to services); (b) filling in the gaps in local responses (e.g., in underserved areas); or (c) offering innovative approaches (e.g., use of mobile telephones for peer support).

- *In concentrated epidemics,* population groups at higher risk of infection, such as FSW and MSM, can be empowered and mobilized to change behavior—a process that has the potential of reducing infections. Policymakers may wish to consider well-focused approaches to support specific, desired outcomes such as those resulting in the removal of access obstacles to prevention and health services by affected population groups.

- *In all cases,* ownership of community responses by their members needs to be fostered and supported, especially in the case of direct donor-funded projects. There is no straight path toward this goal, but funders may want to follow participatory approaches to assess needs, to involve community members in the design of projects to ensure stronger consistency with social customs, and to build the capacity of communities to take over the management of projects or project components supported by normative standards in order to improve quality and results-based contracting schemes. Such participatory approaches would foster a better understanding of the expenditures and the cost of goods, services, and actions. Lack of data on these types of approaches hampers efforts to measure efficiency and effectiveness.

- Implementation of a combination of prevention, biomedical interventions, and/or social support programs would benefit by including specific roles for and expected results from community groups.

- *First, the resulting program would increase the sustainability* of the community response by enabling the program to be supported and promoted by and within the communities.

- *Second, such a program allows community members (such as caregivers) to take on health-related tasks, including peer support or home-based care,* thereby helping to relieve the shortage of health-care professionals in many high-HIV prevalence, low-income countries. However, in this situation the remuneration of caregivers must be considered part of program implementation (UK Consortium 2012).

- *Third, the community response increases the effectiveness of biomedical interventions* that have been shown to be effective, for example, antiretroviral treatment, male circumcision, and the prevention of mother-to-child transmission of HIV, by strengthening social enablers (e.g., stigma reduction, outreach for HIV testing) and program enablers (e.g., retention of patients on antiretroviral therapy, linkages from testing to care) (UNAIDS 2011).

In summary, evidence-informed policy and programming can support community responses to achieve greater effectiveness by (a) improving the targeting of services to the needs of the community, (b) better aligning community-based activities with the HIV epidemic, and (c) strengthening the complementarity between community responses and national programs, such as those for HIV combination prevention measures.

Resource Implications

There is a need to experiment with alternative models of support to the local response. In many cases, the main objective of the support given to civil society was to deliver results (which matter greatly to donors and governments) quickly at the community level. There is now a growing consensus that strengthening the community response itself is essential for longer-term impacts, sustainability, and greater effectiveness of national programs. Implementation of this objective is a long-term endeavor that requires the following:

- *Exploring alternative modes of providing financial support* to the local response, such as conditional cash transfers, which have shown results, or funding mechanisms that are more closely linked to achieving concrete results on the ground, such as performance-based contracting
- *Strengthening national funding channels to facilitate access of community groups and small CBOs to funding*, and improving their technical capacity to collect and report data on expenditures, costs, budgets, and activities. (Ideally, these channels would be more closely linked to government funding mechanisms, which is critical for facilitating the reporting of financial flows and activities and enhancing national ownership.)
- *Providing strong technical support* to community-based activities with standards of practice, normative materials, and links to government agencies
- *Investing in well-defined rather than broad capacity strengthening for project staff and community groups.* (A shift is necessary from fostering generalists to a more specialized approach where community groups are empowered to do better what they already do best—quality—and do more of what they do best when ready.)
- *Better understanding and recognition of the role of caregivers* in general and volunteers in particular (incentives, training), a key resource for CBOs and communities at large

International civil society networks are critical support components of community responses. As the epidemic evolves and the HIV mainstreaming dialogue becomes more prevalent, civil society has an opportunity to inform and be part of this dialogue and influence its outcomes. This might mean that roles and responsibilities of CSOs and networks might need to shift to ensure that the needs of communities are served in a changing fiscal and social environment.

In summary, additional funding envelopes for the community response may or may not be available, but resources for the community response are needed: "no resources, no results." Undoubtedly, it is critical to optimize the resources so that they are used efficiently and effectively. However, issues of efficiency and effectiveness need to be considered along with equity within the context of the places where community groups work. Many are in remote areas, working with disadvantaged, marginalized, and hard-to-reach populations. Issues of equity and consideration of alternatives ("If not with this community mechanism, then with what?") are equally important in the sense that providing services to hard-to-reach populations may involve higher unit costs than those incurred in delivering services to other groups or other geographic areas. Knowing where the epidemic is and where the next 1,000 infections might come from is paramount in determining the direction of strategic investments and programming.

Research Implications

Evaluations of results should be more systematic, not more complex. Adopting such a philosophy would help establish a more continuous process of knowledge building about what works and what does not work, as well as what would help shift investments to areas that would generate greater value for beneficiaries. It could help provide incentives for CBOs and community groups to ensure that tangible benefits are achieved. It would also alert policymakers, program managers, and the communities themselves about changes in the ability of communities to achieve results that benefit the populations they serve and that affect the overall course of the epidemic.

On the thematic front, there are several areas worth pursuing that are common across all community responses:

- *The first would be to examine the evolution of local social capital and the role of volunteers* (including how to sustain their commitment) and the continuum between uncompensated volunteers and fully paid staff. This is an area that might also be influenced by local leadership and commitment, as they are enabling forces for broadening the impacts of community-based activities and their effectiveness.
- *The second would be to examine more closely the issues related to stigma* and the role that real and perceived stigma plays in the access to and use of services by specific population groups. When is access to and use of services hampered, and how much is due to punitive laws, cultural norms, and/or personal fears?
- *Finally, more analytical work is warranted to examine the pathways to achieving results* at the community level, ranging from inputs to impacts of the key programs. The current approach is still a conceptual approach, where program outcome pathways are prepared ex-ante as part of program design. Seldom do programs go back to review and update the outcome pathways based on the empirical experience and knowledge gained by implementing a particular program.

On the methodology front, there is a need to better understand how to apply the most appropriate research methods to examine different aspects of the community response that take into consideration the complexities of evaluating local responses. There is a variety of research methods that can be applied: longitudinal surveys, modeling, household surveys, biomarkers with behavioral change, cost analysis, and others. Each method has its limitations. What is clear is that randomized control trials alone cannot illuminate all aspects of the community response. Creativity coupled with rigor is needed in the selection and application of research methods to examine (a) community-based actions and activities in general and (b) those related particularly to combination prevention, testing, treatment, care, and retention—and the links between the two.

Conclusions

This evaluation provides robust evidence on the contribution of community responses to national HIV and AIDS responses in many cases and circumstances. Nonetheless, there are limitations. This portfolio of studies does not provide a definitive answer to the effects of community responses on knowledge, behavior changes, use of HIV and AIDS services, social changes, and biological outcomes. Intervention-specific studies in selected community contexts would be helpful to corroborate and/or add robustness to the findings where this evaluation found mixed evidence, such as the role of perceived and real stigma in accessing and using services or factors affecting treatment adherence. Thus, the evaluation results do not support a one-size-fits-all design of community responses. However, the findings do indicate that investments have produced results at the community level that do contribute to the desired outcomes of the global response to AIDS. These results point toward a set of implications, as a new generation of local response support emerges.

The findings of this evaluation are supported by and complement other major evaluations such as the recent evaluation of the Avahan program (the India AIDS Initiative of the Bill and Melinda Gates Foundation), which assessed the role of community mobilization and structural interventions in HIV prevention. These two evaluations posit that the behaviors and conditions that promote HIV transmission and access to services are influenced by social norms and values, both at the individual and community levels. Thus, community participation, structural interventions, and organizational development activities coupled with access to services lead to improved outcomes (Rodriguez-García and Bonnel 2012).

In summary, this evaluation supports the appropriateness of considering a mixed-method approach. What is required is a refining of the mixed-method approach to generate more conclusive evidence on more of the areas where community responses can effectively complement national programs: such as in combination with prevention, biomedical intervention, and social action for enabling environments. However, evaluating all aspects of the community response all the time in all countries is not recommended. The critical message here is the importance of building and using robust evidence to support more evidenced-based policies and programs.

Taken individually, each study in this evaluation provides only a partial view of how communities shape the local response to HIV and AIDS. However, when taken in the aggregate, this portfolio of 15 studies provides a robust body of evidence that helps to elucidate and report the effects of community responses in different contexts. This evaluation supports the tenet that investing in communities achieves results that contribute to halting the HIV epidemic.

The community response cannot be taken for granted, nor can it be guaranteed. A certain "community fatigue" could be looming on the horizon, triggered by ever-increasing needs, decreasing resources, and changing priorities. Yet the global HIV goals cannot be achieved without the vital role played by the communities.

Notes

1. Community response is defined as the combination of actions and steps taken by communities, including the provision of goods and services, to prevent and/or address a problem and to bring about social change.

2. Social transformation is defined here as the process by which societal, organizational, and individual change happens, including changes in behaviors or cultural norms and perceptions, as a direct or indirect result of community action.

3. In a concentrated epidemic, HIV has spread among vulnerable groups but is not well established in the general population. In contrast, in a generalized epidemic HIV transmission is mainly outside vulnerable groups. See Wilson (2006) and Denning and DiNenno (2010).

4. See www.aidsconsortium.org.uk for evaluation-related reports and publications.

5. Reference to country and year refers to the study reports of this evaluation and the date of the report. Details of each country study can be found in chapter 5 of this report and in appendix A.

6. Figure O.3 shows CBO density. The density of CBOs was operationalized in Nigeria as the number of CBOs per 100,000 people.

References

Bonnel, R., R. Rodriguez-Garcia, J. Olivier, Q. Wodon, S. McPherson, K. Orr, and J. Ross. 2011. "Funding Mechanisms for the Community Response to HIV and AIDS." Background Paper, World Bank, Washington, DC.

Burkina Faso Evaluation Report. 2011. *Social and Individual Behaviour Change Initiated by Prevention Activities and Antiretroviral Treatment Provision in Burkina Faso.* Washington, DC: World Bank.*

Denning, P., and E. DiNenno. 2010. *Communities in Crisis: Is There a Generalized HIV Epidemic in Impoverished Urban Areas of the United States?* Atlanta: Centers for Disease Control. http://www.cdc.gov/hiv/topics/surveillance/resources/other/poverty .htm.

Global Fund. 2011. *Making a Difference: Results* Report, 2011. Global Fund to Fight AIDS, Tuberculosis and Malaria. Geneva: Global Fund.

Halperin, D. T., O. Mugurungi, T. B, Hallett, B. Muchini, B. Campbell, et al. 2011. "A Surprising Prevention Success: Why Did the HIV Epidemic Decline in Zimbabwe?" *Public Library of Science Medicine* 8: e1000414.

India Evaluation Report. 2011. *Evaluation of Community Mobilization and Empowerment in Relation to HIV Prevention among Female Sex Workers in Karnataka State, South India.* Washington, DC: World Bank.*

————. 2012a. *Using Data to Understand Programmatic Shifts in the Avahan HIV Prevention Program at the Community Level.* Washington, DC: World Bank.*

————. 2012b. *Community Collectivization and Its Association with Selected Outcomes among Female Sex Workers and High-Risk Men Who Have Sex with Men/Transgenders in Andhra Pradesh, India.* Washington, DC: World Bank.*

Kaiser Family Foundation. 2011. *Global Health Interventions: A Review of Evidence.* Washington, DC: Kaiser Family Foundation. www.globalhealth.kff.org/GHIR.aspx.

————. 2012. *Financing the Response to AIDS in Low- and Middle-Income Countries: International Assistance from the G8, European Commission and Other Donor Governments in 2011.* Washington, DC: Kaiser Family Foundation. http://www.kff.org/hivaids/7347.cfm.

Kaiser Family Foundation and UNAIDS. 2012. "Donor Nation Support for HIV Stands Firm but Investments Remain at 2008 Levels." Press Release July 18. http://www.kff.org/hivaids/hiv071812nr.cfm.

Katietek, J. 2012. *Flow of Funds in Community-based Organizations in Kenya, Nigeria and Zimbabwe.* Study Report, World Bank, Washington, DC.

Kenya Evaluation Report. 2011. *Effects of the Community Response on HIV and AIDS in Kenya.* Washington, DC: World Bank.*

Kenya HBCT Evaluation Report. 2012. *The Links between Home-Based HIV Counseling and Testing and HIV Stigma in Western Kenya.* Washington, DC: World Bank.*

Lesotho Evaluation Report. 2011. *Combating the AIDS Pandemic in Lesotho by Understanding Beliefs and Behaviors.* Washington, DC: World Bank.*

Nigeria Evaluation Report. 2011. *Effects of the Community Response to HIV and AIDS in Nigeria.* Washington, DC: World Bank.*

Rodriguez-García, R., R. Bonnel, N. Njie, J. Oliver, B. Pascual, and Q. Wodon. 2011. "Analyzing Community Responses to HIV and AIDS: Operational Framework and Typology." World Bank Policy Research Working Papers 5532, World Bank, Washington, DC.

Rodriguez-García, R., and R. Bonnel. 2012. "Increasing the Evidence Base on the Role of the Community in Response to HIV/AIDS." A commentary in the special supplement of the *Journal of Epidemiology and Community Health.* [*J Epidemiol Community Health 2012;66:Suppl 2 ii7–ii8, doi:10.1136/jech-2012-201298*]

Senegal Evaluation Report. 2010. "HIV/AIDS Sensitization, Social Mobilization and Peer-Mentoring: Evidence from a Randomized Experiment." World Bank, Washington, DC.

South Africa Evaluation Report. 2011. "Timely Peer Adherence and Nutritional Support in Free State Province's Public Sector Antiretroviral Treatment Program." World Bank, Washington, DC.

UK Consortium. 2012. "Past Due: Remuneration and Social Protection for Caregivers in the Context of HIV and AIDS." Policy Brief, London, March. http://aidsconsortium.org.uk/wp-content/uploads/2011/11/UK-AIDS-Consoritum-policy-briefing-remuneration-of-caregivers.pdf.

UNAIDS. 2011. *UNAIDS Strategy 2011–2015: Getting to Zero.* Geneva: UNAIDS.

Wilson, D. 2006. "HIV Epidemiology: A Review of Trends and Lessons." Draft, September 13, World Bank, Washington, DC. http://data.unaids.org/pub/ExternalDocument/2007/20060913wilson_en.pdf.

Zimbabwe Evaluation Report. 2011a. *Social Capital and AIDS Competent Communities: Evidence from Eastern Zimbabwe.* Washington, DC: World Bank.*

———. 2011b. *Evaluation of Community Response to HIV and AIDS: Building Competent Communities: Evidence from Eastern Zimbabwe.* Washington, DC: World Bank.*

———. 2012. *Similarities and Differences in the Community Response to HIV and AIDS in Matabeleland South and Manicaland.* Washington, DC: World Bank.*

*See names of contributors to this report in appendix A

CHAPTER 1

Introduction

Abstract

Chapter 1 is a short introduction that describes the overall context of the evaluation studies, including the available resources for community responses, the role of communities, the need for robust evidence, and the studies that were carried out.

Introduction

The Global AIDS epidemic initially caught the international community unprepared. As epidemiologists struggled to determine the nature of this deadly new disease, and national governments initiated timid official responses, it was the communities of the people affected by the disease who formed the front lines in battling HIV's spread and coming to the aid of those already infected. As international assistance in mitigating the AIDS epidemic scaled up, the community-based response remained a vital force in promoting prevention and providing care. Gradually, significant international funding became available to combat the spread of HIV and help those already suffering from its effects. Recognizing the vital role that the grassroots response played in reaching communities, funders directed some of their assistance to community-based organizations (CBOs) and civil society organizations (CSOs) working within communities. But while other donor-funded programs became subject to increasing scrutiny and pressure to deliver evidence of effectiveness, the community response, due to its diffuse nature, remained difficult to evaluate. As a result, while funding of community organizations continued and monitoring and evaluations were carried out for individual initiatives, the pool of information available for analysis on the subject was substantially narrowed by concerns over poor information quality (Rodriguez-García 2009) and thus, a holistic evaluation of the impact of the community response to HIV remained elusive.

This evaluation aims to fill this gap, to help describe what has been done with the funding committed to community organizations so far, as well as to provide guidance on what the community response can achieve and thus how funders and global NGOs can best engage and leverage this frontline response to the AIDS epidemic in the future.

This evaluation offers a mixed-method approach to measuring the impact of the community response across eight countries, each with unique features that help contribute to a complete understanding of the myriad facets of community responses. We find that community responses can contribute to increased prevention behavior, can multiply the impact of government AIDS programs by increasing uptake of services and can even decrease incidence in some settings. However, its effectiveness depends on the epidemic setting, the approach and intensity of the community groups and other factors. This evaluation provides a roadmap to maximize the impact of community responses through strategic funding and engagement by the international community, to ensure that communities remain a strong pillar of the global AIDS response.

Substantial Investments

In the past decade there has been substantial international commitment to supporting communities and civil society in their efforts to address the AIDS epidemic. During 2003–2009, the four major HIV and AIDS donors combined—the Department for International Development (DfID); the Global Fund to Fight Aids, Tuberculosis and Malaria (Global Fund); the U.S. President's Emergency Plan for AIDS Relief (PEPFAR), and the World Bank—disbursed on average US$690 million per year through CSOs large and small (Bonnel et al. 2011).

The United Kingdom's DfID and the World Bank are among the agencies with an established track record of supporting community-based activities. The British government has long recognized the importance of an active civil society to help relieve poverty. It also recognizes civil society's value in supporting the improvement and quality of lives, especially those of disadvantaged groups and geographical regions, which governments and donors may fail to reach.

The World Bank supports a significant number of community-based efforts around the globe. In the area of community-driven development alone, the World Bank currently supports more than 400 projects in 95 countries, valued at almost US$30 billion.[1] Regarding the HIV epidemic, the World Bank pioneered a multisectoral approach to increase access to HIV prevention, care, and treatment programs, with an emphasis on encouraging local responses. By the late 1990s, the Multi-Country HIV/AIDS Program (MAP) provided one of the first funding mechanisms at the global level for HIV/AIDS. An estimated US$2.4 billion was disbursed for all World Bank HIV/AIDS projects in 2003–2010. Thirty-nine percent of these funds were committed to the local response, amounting to the largest percentage by allocation.

PEPFAR provided the largest funding for HIV and AIDS: US$12.4 billion in 2003–10. On average, it is estimated that national (as opposed to international) CSOs received about US$7.4 billion during this period. Similarly, the Global Fund disbursed US$6.1 billion from 2003 to mid-2010, of which an estimated US$1.1 billion was made available to CSOs.

Despite this level of commitment, it has been difficult to demonstrate outcomes from global investments in the local response to HIV and AIDS. A review of the effectiveness of World Bank HIV assistance conducted in 2005 by the World Bank's Independent Evaluation Group (IEG) (formally the Operations Evaluation Department, or OED) underscored the need to improve the evidence base for decision making—and more specifically to rigorously evaluate community-driven HIV activities (World Bank 2005).

Diverse Roles of Communities

Communities play different roles in different HIV epidemics. In terms of concentrated epidemics,[2] many studies across the world have indicated that peer-led targeted prevention interventions result in increased knowledge as well as decreased prevalence of sexually transmitted infections (STIs) among groups at high risk of infection (Rou et al. 2007). Successes have been especially widespread for community responses to HIV in commercial sex work. Effective prevention interventions for men who have sex with men (MSM) and injecting drug users (IDUs) have also been reported, but further progress depends on the development of innovative strategies to address what for many are repressive environments.

Thus, many studies recommend that prevention programs address the complex social, cultural, and economic vulnerabilities faced by groups at high risk of infection. Indeed, there has been widespread endorsement of empowerment as part of such community mobilization, making it a core principal of many national AIDS plans (Evans, Jana, and Lambert 2010). The evidence from this evaluation supports this recommendation.

In terms of generalized HIV epidemics, community roles are different. In southern African countries where the generalized epidemics have reached exceptionally high prevalence rates, very large numbers of people are living with HIV.[3] In such a context, communities have taken on wide-ranging tasks that cover the whole spectrum of interventions from prevention to care, support, and mitigation.

Although a number of studies report the effects of microlevel initiatives, there remains little robust evidence concerning the pathways through which community mobilization can reverse the course of an HIV epidemic. A randomized control trial of adherence to treatment supported by this evaluation may be able to address this issue, studying the extent to which peer support increases treatment adherence. To the extent that treatment can prevent HIV infections, then it could be shown that community intervention could contribute to halting the epidemic. This is supported by the 2011 UNAIDS Issues Brief: "A new investment framework for the global HIV response," which places community mobilization as a key for sound investments (Schwartlander et al. 2011).

In countries with lower levels of HIV prevalence, the HIV epidemic is often "mixed," in the sense that it may include features of a concentrated epidemic in some areas and a generalized epidemic in others. These characteristics have often been overlooked in the expansion of community responses. AIDS programs in these areas were often designed to fund the same type of community mobilization as in high HIV prevalence countries. More recent prevention guidelines envisage a much more limited role for communities, where communities engage in key activities aligned to the characteristics of these epidemics (UNAIDS 2007). The evidence from this evaluation supports this approach of a more targeted and focused role for communities in this context. It also identifies areas where community responses can have an impact as well as areas where the potential for impact is less clear.

Communities and Government Programs

Communities and their organizations increasingly provide a wide range of HIV and AIDS services and often broader social and health-related services. Some of these activities represent normal coping mechanisms of the communities that became highlighted as the communities became severely affected by the epidemic. These include, among other things, providing home-based care and support for people affected and infected by HIV, creating support groups for people living with HIV, and helping families cope with AIDS orphans.

However, there are other activities that have been initiated in response to the availability of donor funding or because of a lack of government services. This has raised questions as to whether these activities generate value for money, and whether they should be provided by government ministries or agencies as part of the national response rather than by the communities. That conversation will continue, but currently in most countries the community response is one of the key pillars of the national strategic plan. Further clarification of and support for leveraging community groups and their activities would contribute to better results and efficiencies.

Need for Evidence

Having a stronger evidence base would help policy makers plan and implement a more effective HIV response at the community level. This need is reflected in DfID's 2011 strategy titled *Towards Zero Infections: The UK's Position Paper on HIV in the Developing World*, which sets as a priority the need to "increase . . . investment in rigorous evaluations to really understand what works for prevention and promulgating it" with the objective of "developing an approach that considers the structural drivers of the epidemic beyond biomedical and behavioral interventions" (DfID 2011).

The evidence generated by this evaluation offers a number of benefits for the targeting of global and national investments. It provides evidence in support of strengthening the critical enablers of the UNAIDS investment framework for basic program activities (PMTCT, condom promotion and distribution, outreach activities for groups at high risk of infection (FSWs and MSM), treatment and care, support, and behavior change), and for improving social enablers in the areas of stigmatization and gender/domestic abuse.

Using this evidence can be helpful to countries preparing evidence-based funding proposals for the Global Fund, as well. It would also help other development partners, such as USAID or PEPFAR, in their efforts to support local involvement in their HIV and AIDS programs. The 2011 PEPFAR guidance for the prevention of STIs outlines an increased role for communities, especially with respect to behavioral interventions, but more broadly as a tool for increasing the demand for biomedical services such as HIV counseling and testing (HCT) and voluntary male circumcision.

At the country level, the data collected by specific evaluations can provide a baseline for evaluating the community pillar of national HIV strategies or for carrying out a program review. Identification of the areas where the community response is effective would inform the allocation of resources, suggest areas where greater coordination of activities with government services would be beneficial, and help identify specific technical assistance needs. Finally, national researchers might find the approach used in this evaluation particularly useful as it opens up new possibilities for evidence building.

Given this body of evidence, then, what seem to be the key features of successful community responses?

Evaluating the Community Response

The empirical studies conducted as part of the *Evaluation of the Community Response to HIV and AIDS*—a foundation of this report, conducted between 2009 and 2012 in partnership with DfID and the UK Consortium on AIDS and International Development, and presented here—are meant to complement previous research efforts and to provide policy guidance. The evaluation makes important arguments for the optimization of HIV and AIDS responses at a time when financial resources remain flat. It also comes at a time when major donors are emphasizing the importance of strengthening community systems (Global Fund), local ownership (PEPFAR), and investment in community mobilization (Joint United Nations Programme on HIV/AIDS—UNAIDS).

This document synthesizes and analyzes findings from 17 analytical studies, including 11 evaluations carried out in 8 countries. Taken in isolation, each study of this evaluation provides only partial information on one or several aspects of community responses to HIV and AIDS. Taken together, however, these studies provide a body of evidence on the holistic effects of the response and rate the generally positive effects of the community response to HIV in different contexts. Moreover, this compendium of evidence presents a path

Table 1.1 Summary of Studies

Country	Topic	Method
Burkina Faso	Impact of community prevention activities on knowledge, prevention behavior, and stigma	Quasi-experimental
India (Karnataka)	Impact of mobilization and empowerment among female sex workers	Quasi-experimental and qualitative
India (Andhra Pradesh)	Impact of community collectivization among female sex workers and high-risk men	Quasi-experimental

table continues next page

Table 1.1 Summary of Studies (continued)

Country	Topic	Method
Kenya	Understand funding and activities of CBOs and evaluating the impact of strong community response on knowledge, behavior, and service uptake	Quasi-experimental (matching) and qualitative
Kenya (HBCT)	Ability to implement home-based testing in presence of stigma and impact of testing effort on community leader and member stigma	Randomized controlled trial
Lesotho	Relationship between HIV/AIDS stigma and take-up of services/testing in a high-prevalence area	Analytical
Nigeria	Understand funding and activities of CBOs and evaluating the impact of strong community response on knowledge, behavior, and service uptake	Quasi-experimental, analytical, and qualitative
Senegal	Impact of social mobilization on counseling and testing uptake (comparing peer mentoring to traditional sensitization)	Randomized controlled trial
South Africa	Impact of peer support and nutrition supplementation on treatment adherence	Randomized controlled trial
Zimbabwe	Impact of grassroots community group membership on behavior, service utilization, and HIV incidence	Quasi-experimental (longitudinal)

Analytical and desk studies

Typology of community response

Cost structure of CBOs budgets in Kenya

Funding mechanisms

OVC review

Analysis of CBOs resources and expenditures in Kenya, Nigeria, and Zimbabwe

Note: Some listed studies contain multiple analytical pieces such as Nigeria where a state-by-state analysis was done after the evaluation was completed. This makes up the 17 studies. Chapter 2 details the approach and methodology of this multicounty evaluation and summarizes the objectives of the evaluation. The approaches are described in more detail in appendix C. Chapter 3 presents findings related to the capacity of CBOs and their overall resources, then focuses on the resulting impacts. Chapter 4 presents an overview of the eight country evaluation studies describing the types of community responses evaluated and the main results. Chapter 5 outlines the features of successful community responses and their variances across settings. Conclusions and recommendations are presented in chapter 6. AIDS = acquired immune deficiency syndrome, CBO = community-based organization, HBCT = home-based counseling and testing, HIV = human immunodeficiency virus, OVC = orphans and vulnerable children.

forward for aid workers, policy makers, and researchers on leveraging and engaging with communities and better understanding community responses. The included studies are summarized in table 1.1.

Notes

1. "What Have Been the Impacts of World Bank Community-Driven Development (CDD) Programs?" April 2012. Internal draft paper prepared by the Social Protection Unit, World Bank.

2. Concentrated epidemics are those where the transmission of infections are largely limited to sex workers (SW), men who have sex with men (MSM), and injecting drug

users (IDUs). Such epidemics could be interrupted by effective SW, MSM, and IDU interventions.

3. Generalized epidemics are epidemics in which the transmission of infections takes place largely in the general population, and would persist despite effective SW, MSM and IDU interventions.

References

Bonnel, R., R. Rodriguez-Garcia, J. Olivier, Q. Wodon, S. McPherson, K. Orr, and J. Ross. 2011. "Funding Mechanisms for the Community Response to HIV and AIDS." Background Paper, World Bank, Washington, DC.

DfID (UK Department for International Development). 2011. "Towards Zero Infections: The UK's Position Paper on HIV in the Developing World." UK DfID, London.

Evans, C., S. Jana, and H. Lambert. 2010. "What Makes a Structural Intervention? Reducing Vulnerability to HIV in Community Settings, with Particular Reference to Sex Work." *Global Public Health* 595: 449–61.

PEPFAR (The US President's Emergency Plan for AIDS Relief). 2011. *Guidance for the Prevention of Sexually Transmitted HIV Infections.* Washington, DC: PEPFAR.

Rodriguez-García, R. 2009. "Evaluating the Community Response to HIV/AIDS." *World Bank Development Dialogue Notes 1*, no. 2. World Bank, Washington, DC.

Rou, K., Z. Wu, S. G. Sullivan, F. Li, J. Guan, C. Xu, W. Liu, D. Liu, and Y. Yin. 2007. "A Five-City Trial of a Behavioural Intervention to Reduce Sexually Transmitted Disease/ HIV Risk among Sex Workers in China." *AIDS* 21(Suppl 8): S95–101.

Schwartlander, B., J. Stover, T. Hallett, R. Atun, C. Avila, E. Gouws, M. Bartos, P. Ghys, M. Opuni, D. Barr, B. lsallaq, L. Bollinger, M. de Freitas, G. Garnett, C. Holmes, K. Legins, Y. Pillay, E. Anderson, C. McClure, G. Hirnschall, M. Laga, and N. Padian. 2011. "Towards an Improved Investment Approach for an Effective Response to HIV/ AIDS." *Lancet* 337: 2031–41.

UNAIDS (Joint United Nations Programme on HIV/AIDS). 2007. *Practical Guidelines for Intensifying HIV Prevention: Towards Universal Access.* Geneva: UNAIDS.

World Bank. 2005. *Committing to Results: Improving the Effectiveness of HIV/AIDS Assistance.* Washington, DC: World Bank.

Approach and Methodology

Abstract

Chapter 2 indicates how the evaluation of community responses was designed and carried out. It describes the typology challenge created by the diversity of communities and the diversity of community responses. It discusses the mixed-method approach that was used for the evaluation studies, their components (randomized controlled trials, quasi-experimental studies, longitudinal studies, qualitative studies, analysis of local organizations' budgets, and analytical studies), and their areas of investigation.

Introduction

Chapter 2 details the approach and methodology of this multicountry evaluation. More detailed information is included in appendix C.

Objectives

This evaluation aimed to generate knowledge on the local response to HIV and AIDS. The purpose of the evaluation was to (a) report HIV and AIDS results achieved at the community level, (b) identify areas where investments can achieve greater results, and (c) discuss critical policy and programmatic issues.

More specifically, this evaluation examined broad community-based activities, services, and actions; specific interventions; and the flow of funds at the global and community levels. It applies a definition of community understood in terms of identity (men who have sex with men (MSM) and sex workers (SW), for instance) as well as a community defined in terms of geographic location.

Using the hypothesis that the community response leads to community-based results, and adds value to the national response, specific research questions were selected based on the causal-logic theory of change model: that is, studying how and why an initiative works, looking for changes in knowledge, behaviors, practices, coverage, utilization of services, and HIV and AIDS-related health outcomes along the continuum of prevention, treatment, care, support, and mitigation. Quantitative, qualitative, and financial data were collected and analyzed to provide a better understanding of the nuances of the findings.

One shortcoming of some earlier evaluations is that they focused on narrow evaluations of broad programs or projects. They did not go far enough in explaining what benefits accrued to communities and households by the combination of activities at the community level. This evaluation aims to fill this void by providing robust data on outcomes and impacts and examining possible explanatory factors that may affect the results.

What Is the Community Response?

"Community response" *refers to the combination of actions and steps taken by communities for the public good, including the provision of goods and services* (see box 2.1). Since the beginning of the HIV epidemic, community groups have been at the front lines of country HIV responses. Community groups mobilized public action, thereby laying the foundation for the establishment of national responses with support from their governments, the scientific community, and public health authorities (Berkman et al. 2005; UNAIDS 2006; Zuniga 2006). In many countries, community-based organizations (CBOs) were the pioneers of counseling and home-based care for the sick (Roberts, Hickey, and Rosner 2006; UNAIDS 2006).

The role of communities in national responses received a major boost from the 2001 United Nations General Assembly Special Session on HIV/AIDS (UNGASS). UNGASS galvanized donors and political leaders to implement a multisectoral response involving national AIDS commissions, government ministries, and CSOs. Since then, community responses have become an integral part

---

Box 2.1 Definitions

Communities can be described as the following:

• Those sharing a *cultural identity* (members belong to a group that shares common characteristics or interests), such as people living with HIV and AIDS, MSM, and SW.
• Those sharing a *geographic sense of place* (a group in a location or an administrative entity). For instance, in Kenya, the Ministry of Medical Services defines community as

a collection of household units brought together by common interests, and/or made up of at least 5,000 people (or 100 households) living in the same geographical area. These villages are mainly administered by a chief based at the location level. A collection of villages formed a sub-location, which then collect to form a location. A community would share, therefore, similar culture, social practices, beliefs, and value systems.

The *community response* can be defined as follows:

• The combination of actions and steps taken by communities, including the provision of goods and services, to prevent and/or address a problem to bring about social change.

Source: Rodriguez-García et al. 2011.

---

of nearly all national HIV and AIDS strategies. However, what community response means has been a source of confusion, as it has been interpreted in various ways. To address this issue, a typology of community responses and an operational framework for analyzing them were developed for this evaluation (see Rodriguez-García et al. 2011).

Communities: The Typology Challenge

Communities are intrinsically heterogeneous. One way they can be defined is by their cultural identity, in which case a community is defined by a group of people who have some commonality. Examples include people belonging to a church group, groups of people living with HIV, SW, or MSM. This cultural identity definition was used for evaluating the community response in India. Communities can also refer to groups of people linked by virtue of living in the same geographical place such as a village or a town. This definition was used for evaluating the community response in Kenya, Nigeria, and Zimbabwe (see box 2.1).

Communities can also be classified by their degree of formality. At the most informal levels are households and indigenous grassroots groups. These groups are more or less active based on need (e.g., church groups, burial societies, and AIDS groups). At a slightly more formal level are CBOs. At the most formal levels are nongovernmental organization (NGOs) and faith-based organizations (FBOs). Both the qualitative and the quantitative analyses of community responses revealed institutional differences between CBOs and NGOs (see figure 2.1).

CBOs tend to be community driven and work within the communities they represent. They reflect local ways of forming groups and interacting with local leaders (such as traditional chiefs in Africa), and they draw upon local resources.

Figure 2.1 Dimensions of the Community Response Analyzed in the Country Evaluations

	Burkina Faso	Kenya HBCT	India	Kenya, Nigeria	Lesotho	Senegal	South Africa	Zimbabwe
Most informal	↑	↑	↑	↑	↑	↑	↑	↑
Households	●	●		●	●		●	
Community initiatives			●					●
CBOs/FBOs		●	●	●		●		●
NGOs								
Most formal	↓	↓	↓	↓	↓	↓	↓	↓

Sources: Burkina Faso Evaluation Report 2011; India Evaluation Report 2011, 2012a, 2012b; Kenya Evaluation Report 2011; Kenya HBCT Evaluation Report 2012; Lesotho Evaluation Report 2011; Nigeria Evaluation Report 2011; Senegal Evaluation Report 2010; South Africa Evaluation Report 2011; Zimbabwe Evaluation Report 2011a, 2011b, 2012.
Note: CBO = community-based organization, FBO = faith-based organization, HBCT = home-based counseling and testing, NGO = nongovernmental organization.

CBOs are typically small; sometimes they may not employ permanent staff, but rely instead on large numbers of volunteers to fulfill their mission and/or to deliver services. In contrast, NGOs and FBOs may deliver various services to local communities as implementers of donor- or government-funded programs. They are usually larger than CBOs and have a more formal institutional structure that helps them to meet the various fiduciary, reporting, and monitoring requirements of their funders.

To capture the diversity of communities, the country evaluations looked at different types of entities. In Burkina Faso, the focus was on households. In India, communities of SWs, MSM, and transgender individuals were the subjects of two evaluations. In Zimbabwe, the focus was on grassroots organizations (rotating credit clubs, farmers' associations, youth clubs, and so on) that constituted different communities. In Kenya and Nigeria, the evaluation looked at CBO activities in their catchment areas (see figure 2.1).

The activities carried out by community organizations vary across countries. An example of CBO activities in the case of Kenya and Nigeria is presented in table 2.1. In Kenya, CBOs were engaged mainly in increasing the awareness and knowledge of HIV and AIDS and in behavior change; providing support for people living with HIV and AIDS (PLWHA) (for instance, by the training of home-caregivers and facilitating rotating credit associations and income-generating activities); and carrying out activities targeting orphans and vulnerable children (OVC) through payment of school fees and buying school supplies and uniforms. Other activities such as condom distribution, promotion of HIV counseling and testing (HCT), referrals to health clinics, and provision of treatment were carried out by only a few CBOs. A different pattern of activities emerged from the surveyed CBOs in Nigeria. Although these organizations were also engaged in prevention, they were more active in providing various services (e.g., treatment and support to people living with HIV and to OVC).

A Mixed-Method Approach

Progress in generating robust evidence on the community response to HIV and AIDS has been hampered by various methodological difficulties. Randomized controlled trials (RCTs) are usually viewed as the gold standard for research designs. They are well adapted for clinical trials but not so well for evaluating the impact of prevention or behavioral interventions that may be implemented by various actors with multiple results. This conclusion emerged from a systematic review of 49 RCTs for the prevention of the sexual transmission of HIV covering the period from 1987 to 2009 (Padian et al. 2010).[1]

Among the nine RCT evaluations concerning the community response, only one (for sexually transmitted infections (STIs) treatment) was found to be effective; more recent clinical trials have thrown considerable doubt as to the effectiveness of this research design (Celum et al. 2010). In total, only seven trials provided robust evidence about six interventions (microbicides, STI treatment, male circumcision–male acquisition, HIV treatment as prevention, PMTCT, and

Table 2.1 Activity Areas and Number of CBOs per Area in Kenya and Nigeria

	Kenya (27 surveyed CBOs)	Nigeria (69 surveyed CBOs)
Prevention	EIC (18)	EIC (38)
		Advocacy (meetings) (13)
	Speaking at Barazas (public meeting place) (10)	Public lectures (7)
	BCC (16)	BCC (2)
	Condom distribution (3)	Condom distribution (16)
	Hosting HCT (2)	HCT (9)
	Promotion of HCT (2)	HCT referral (7)
		Others: abstinence promotion, peer education, community theater, health education
Treatment	Treatment provision (2)	Provision of medication (3)
		Opportunistic infections treatment (4)
	Treatment referral (2)	Treatment referral (3)
Support	Provision of food and toiletries (8)	Financial support (17)
		Material support (6)
		Psychological support (12)
		Referral services (3)
		Burial services (1)
Care	Training of caregivers (5)	HBC (9)
		HBC training (3)
		HBC supplies (2)
		Visiting the sick (5)
Impact mitigation	Rotating credit associations (3)	Communal farming (4)
	Income generating activities (3)	Income-generating activity (8)
		Microcredit (6)
		Legal support (2)
OVC support	Paying/supplementing school fees (9)	School fees (14)
	Buying school supplies (6)	School materials (12)
	Buying school uniforms (2)	Psychological support (9)
		Referral to services (6)

Source: Compiled by the authors for this report.
Note: BCC = behavior change communication; EIC = education, information and communication; HBC = home-based care; HCT = HIV counseling and testing; OVC = orphans and vulnerable children.

pre-exposure prophylaxis). Almost 90 percent of the reviewed trials were "flat." In other words, they were unable to demonstrate either a positive or adverse effect, a result that is attributable mainly to trial design and implementation. A common issue is the reduced statistical power of these evaluations, resulting from a lower than expected HIV incidence. Another issue is that some interventions overlapped between the treatment group and the control group, which made it difficult to detect a statistically different effect between the two groups.

Not only are there difficulties in measurement when using RCTs, but there are also challenges in manipulating a treatment that is by its nature organic—that is, one cannot randomize the community response, because effective community response is driven by and derives from the community. In these cases, RCT cannot be applied to isolated individuals or particular areas such as a medical intervention but rather must be woven into the fabric of the community. Therefore,

RCTs are inherently not well designed to deal with the types of community responses most likely to have an impact. RCTs are appropriate in other cases, and were applied for specific interventions in this evaluation.

This evaluation has collected substantial and wide-ranging field data, mostly primary data—quantitative, qualitative, and financial. In some instances, primary data were complemented by new analysis of secondary data. Given the vast range and variety of community responses, this evaluation applied a mixed-method, multicountry, portfolio approach, implemented by multidisciplinary teams of researchers.

The design of the evaluation involved several phases. In the first, the concept note was reviewed in the context of a broad consultative process involving various experts, international agencies, donor agencies, and civil society organizations that took place in 2008 (figure 2.2). The design of the evaluation was further revised in 2009 during the second phase. Several studies helped inform the evaluation and the protocol that was developed. Country evaluations started in 2010 and continued throughout 2011. They were accompanied by additional studies on specific topics that country evaluations had revealed as important for community responses, such as funding of CBOs and the role of volunteers. All studies collected primary data. Final triangulation, analysis, and dissemination of results started in 2012.

To address some of these methodological issues and the highly contextual nature of community-level work, the evaluation used a mixed-method, multicountry approach, while preserving the rigor of the exercise (see appendix C for more detail). It considered several research designs (experimental, quasi-

Figure 2.2 Design and Implementation of the Evaluation: A Phase-In Approach

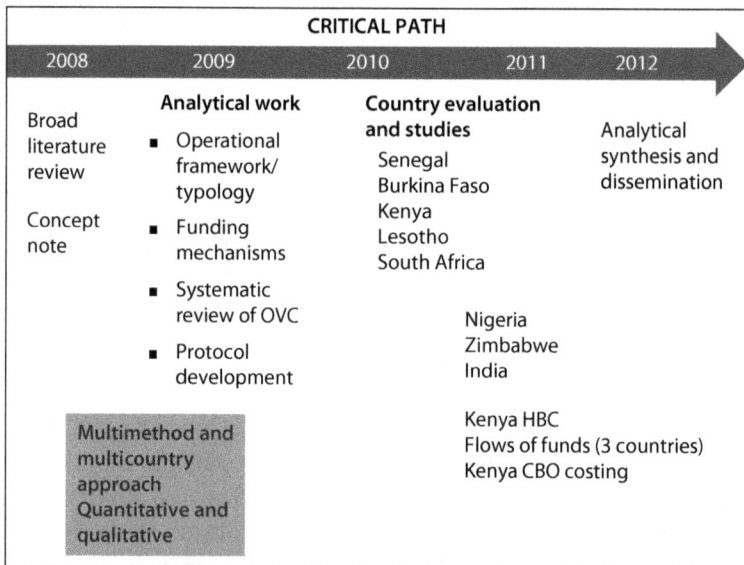

Note: CBO = community-based organization, HBC = home-based care, OVC = orphans and vulnerable children.

experimental, longitudinal); collected quantitative, qualitative, and financial data; applied several data collection instruments (surveys, key informant interviews, budget reviews); and involved multidisciplinary teams of researchers. In a mixed-method approach, methods compensate for each other's weaknesses, providing more coherent, reliable, and useful information from which to draw conclusions. The approach is often considered superior to using single methods. Thus, in this mixed-method approach, triangulation becomes a central function used to see how data sets confirm, challenge, or explain the findings (World Bank 2012, chapter 11).

To provide corroborating evidence, the evaluations were chosen so that the same type of intervention would be studied in several countries, and different sources of information would be used to corroborate the results of the evaluations. In cases where an intervention was found to be associated with the same result in another country, the overall evidence that this intervention could be causally linked to the findings became stronger.

Six evaluations (Burkina Faso, Kenya, Nigeria, Zimbabwe, and two in India) followed a quasi-experimental design, and three evaluations (Kenya Home-Based Counseling and Testing [HBCT], Senegal, and South Africa) used an experimental design with a randomization of the groups being studied and division into control and comparison groups (see table C.1 in appendix C). Although some believe that quasi-experimental designs can show only whether or not there is an association between the studied interventions and the outcomes, others believe it can also show causation. In contrast, RCTs can indicate whether there is, in fact, a causal relationship. However, their application is generally limited to evaluating the effects of specific interventions rather than the results of a broad package of activities, such as those in a community response. The experimental and quasi-experimental studies used robust methods for establishing a "counterfactual," meaning: What would have happened to a similar group of people in the absence of community intervention?

Further explanation for the observed results was obtained from other sources of information. These included qualitative analysis of the role of communities provided by surveys and in-depth interviews of community members, community groups, CBOs, and key informants (India, Kenya, Nigeria, and Zimbabwe); analysis of CBO resources and expenditures (Kenya, Nigeria, and Zimbabwe); and other specific background and desk studies. By triangulating quantitative data with qualitative data and analysis of funding, the country evaluations that followed quasi-experimental methods were able to report the pathways through which the community responses operate. This builds a convincing body of evidence.

The working principles of the evaluation recognize some of the limitations of the methodology. In theory, it would have been preferable to study all the aspects of the community response in every country affected by the HIV epidemic. In practice, this was not possible or desirable, as the logistical implications would have been overwhelming. Instead, the chosen approach was to evaluate a number of community responses that would be representative of the different types of responses and the various settings in which they play a large role in the overall HIV/AIDS response. The difficulty involved in evaluating a complex set of activities with various dimensions such as the community response is another challenge. To address it, the country evaluations relied on a combination of studies that shed light on different aspects of community responses.

Nevertheless, the evaluation does not provide a definitive or one-size-fits-all answer to the question of whether community responses affect knowledge, behavior changes, social transformation, access to services, and biological outcomes. Given the context-specific nature of the evaluation studies, findings may not be readily generalized to other countries. Finally, it is important to keep in mind that the evaluation does not indicate whether the various types of community responses are cost effective. Intervention-specific cost analyses would have to be carried out to answer that question.

Conceptual Framework of Community Responses

Figure 2.3 illustrates a causal-logic theory of change. It provides a linear view of what is really a complex web of assumptions about actions undertaken to transform inputs into outputs, outcomes, and ultimately impacts. This figure presents a simplified theory of change to help understand the cause-effect theory that guided the design of the evaluation. A more complete formulation that takes into account other factors in the theory of change is presented in appendix C.

The areas of investigation are summarized in table 2.2 according to the causal-logic theory, detailing inputs, activities, outputs, outcomes, and impact.

Figure 2.3 A Causal-Logic Theory of Change Linking the Community Response to Improved HIV and AIDS-Related Results

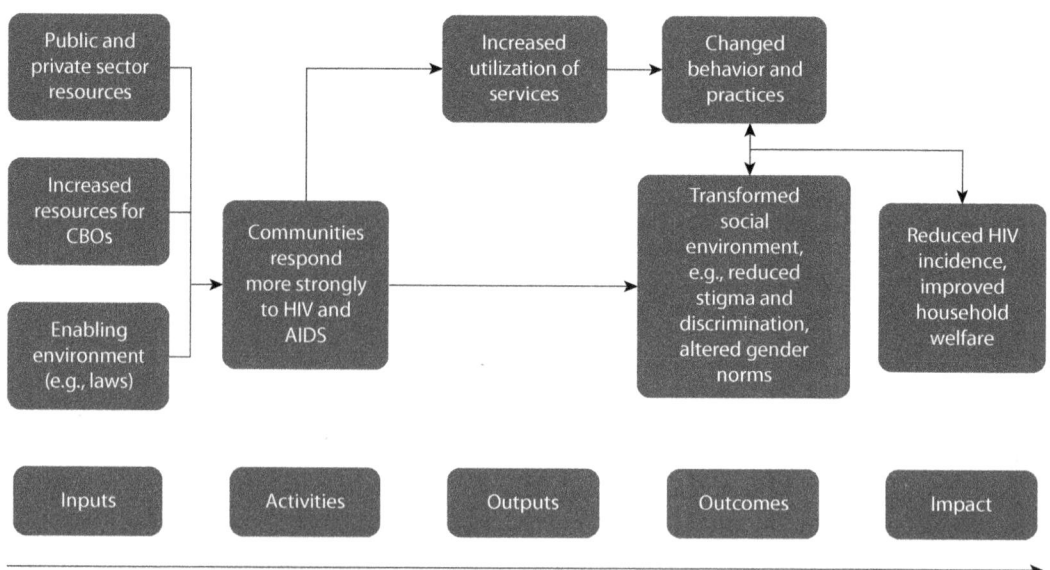

Note: AIDS = acquired immune deficiency syndrome, CBO = community-based organization, HIV = human immunodeficiency virus.

Table 2.2 Main Areas Examined by Each Study

Study	Inputs	Activities	Outputs	Outcomes	Impact
Burkina Faso	—	—	Drivers of participation in prevention activities; Role in service utilization	Effect of participation on knowledge, risk, and stigma	—
India FSW (Karnataka)	—	—	Effect of community mobilization on high-risk groups	Effect of community mobilization on empowerment, service use, and risk	Impact of mobilization on STI prevalence
India FSW; MSM (Andra Pradesh)	—	—	Relationship between community collectivization and service utilization	Effect of community collectivization on risk and self-efficacy	—
Kenya	Funding sources and allocation	Activities engaged in by CBOs	Effect on service utilization	Effect on knowledge, awareness, behavior, and social transformation	—
Kenya HBCT	—	—	Role of communities and leaders in impacting service uptake	Effect on knowledge, behavior, testing, and stigma	—
Lesotho	—	—	Impact of stigma on uptake of testing	—	—
Nigeria	Funding sources and allocation	Activities engaged in by CBOs	Effect on service utilization	Effect on knowledge, awareness, behavior, and social transformation	—
Senegal	—	Effectiveness of types of engagement	Result of strategies on influencing testing and counseling uptake	Effect on risk behavior	—
South Africa	—	—	—	Effect of peer support and nutritional supplement on treatment adherence	—
Zimbabwe	Funding sources and allocations	—	Effect of grassroots membership on service utilization	Effect of community involvement on risk behaviors	Impact on HIV incidence

Sources: Burkina Faso Evaluation Report 2011; India Evaluation Report 2011, 2012a, 2012b; Kenya Evaluation Report 2011; Kenya HBCT Evaluation Report 2012; Lesotho Evaluation Report 2011; Nigeria Evaluation Report 2011; Senegal Evaluation Report 2010; South Africa Evaluation Report 2011; Zimbabwe Evaluation Report 2011a, 2011b, 2012.

Note: CBO = community-based organization, FSW = female sex workers, HBCT = home-based counseling and testing, HIV = human immunodeficiency virus, MSM = men who have sex with men, STI = sexually transmitted infection.

— = not studied.

Note

1. Eligible evaluations in that study were those that used RCTs, evaluated interventions to prevent sexual transmission in nonpregnant populations, and reported HIV incidence as the primary or secondary outcome.

References

Berkman, A., J. Garcia, M. Munoz-Laboy, V. Paiva, and R. Parker. 2005. "A Critical Analysis of the Brazilian Response to HIV/AIDS: Lessons Learned for Controlling and Mitigating the Epidemic in Developing Countries." *American Journal of Public Health* 95 (7): 1162–72.

Burkina Faso Evaluation Report. 2011. *Social and Individual Behaviour Change Initiated by Prevention Activities and Antiretroviral Treatment Provision in Burkina Faso.* Washington, DC: World Bank.*

Celum, C., A. Wald, J. R. Lingappa, A. S. Magaret, R. S. Wang, N. Mugo, A. Mujugira, et al. 2010. "Acyclovir and Transmission of HIV-1 from Persons Infected with HIV-1 and HSV-2. *N Engl J Med* 362: 427–39.

India Evaluation Report. 2011. *Evaluation of Community Mobilization and Empowerment in Relation to HIV Prevention among Female Sex Workers in Karnataka State, South India.* Washington, DC: World Bank.*

———. 2012a. *Using Data to Understand Programmatic Shifts in the Avahan HIV Prevention Program at the Community Level.* Washington, DC: World Bank.*

———. 2012b. *Community Collectivization and Its Association with Selected Outcomes among Female Sex Workers and High-Risk Men Who Have Sex with Men/Transgenders in Andhra Pradesh, India.* Washington, DC: World Bank.*

Kenya Evaluation Report. 2011. *Effects of the Community Response on HIV and AIDS in Kenya.* Washington, DC: World Bank.*

Kenya HBCT Evaluation Report. 2012. *The Links between Home-Based HIV Counseling and Testing and HIV Stigma in Western Kenya.* Washington, DC: World Bank.*

Lesotho Evaluation Report. 2011. *Combating the AIDS Pandemic in Lesotho by Understanding Beliefs and Behaviors.* Washington, DC: World Bank.*

Nigeria Evaluation Report 2011. *Effects of the Community Response to HIV and AIDS in Nigeria.* Washington, DC: World Bank.*

Padian, N. S., S. I. McCoy, J. E. Balkus, and J. N. Wasserheit. 2010. "Weighing the Gold in the Gold Standard: Challenges in HIV Prevention Research." *AIDS* 24: 621–35.

Roberts, R., A. Hickey, and Z. Rosner. 2006. "The Role of Community Involvement in HIV Programmes in South Africa." In *The HIV Pandemic: Local and Global Implications*, ed. J. Beck, N. Mays, A. Whiteside, and J. Zuniga, 721–33. Oxford: Oxford University Press.

Rodriguez-García, R., R. Bonnel, N. Njie, J. Oliver, B. Pascual, and Q. Wodon. 2011. "Analyzing Community Responses to HIV and AIDS: Operational Framework and Typology." World Bank Policy Research Working Papers 5532, World Bank, Washington, DC.

Senegal Evaluation Report. 2010. *HIV/AIDS Sensitization, Social Mobilization and Peer-Mentoring: Evidence from a Randomized Experiment.* Washington, DC: World Bank.*

South Africa Evaluation Report. 2011. *Timely Peer Adherence and Nutritional Support in Free State Province's Public Sector Antiretroviral Treatment Program*. Washington, DC: World Bank.*

UNAIDS (Joint United Nations Programme on HIV/AIDS). 2006. *The Essential Role of Civil Society*. Report on the Global AIDS Epidemic. A UNAIDS 10th Anniversary Special Edition. Geneva: UNAIDS.

World Bank. 2012. *Building Better Policies: The Nuts and Bolts of Monitoring and Evaluation Systems*. ed. G. Lopez-Acevedo, P. Krause, and K. MacKay. Washington, DC: World Bank.

Zimbabwe Evaluation Report. 2011a. *Social Capital and AIDS Competent Communities: Evidence from Eastern Zimbabwe*. Washington, DC: World Bank.*

———. 2011b. *Evaluation of Community Response to HIV and AIDS: Building Competent Communities: Evidence from Eastern Zimbabwe*. Washington, DC: World Bank.*

———. 2012. *Similarities and Differences in the Community Response to HIV and AIDS in Matabeleland South and Manicaland*. Washington, DC: World Bank.*

Zuniga, J. 2006. "The Contribution of Civil Society." In *The HIV Pandemic: Local and Global Implications*, ed. J. Beck, N. Mays, A. Whiteside, and J. Zuniga, 707–19. Oxford: Oxford University Press.

---

*See names of contributors to this report in appendix A.

Key Findings and Cross-Cutting Issues

Abstract

Chapter 3 addresses the questions of what the available resources for community responses are and whether they have generated tangible results at the community level. The first section of the chapter therefore focuses on resources, including those made available by donors and those mobilized by Community-Based Organizations themselves. The second section describes the resulting impacts of community responses on knowledge about HIV and AIDS, risk behaviors, access and use of HIV and AIDS services, social transformation (e.g., gender, stigma, social cohesion) and AIDS-related health outcomes.

Introduction

An underlying concern with community responses relates to a fundamental question: do communities have the capacity to effect genuine and long-lasting change? One would expect the overall impact to be small if the resources available to community-based organizations (CBOs) are limited. One objective of this chapter, then, is to present findings related to the capacity of CBOs and their overall resources. The first section of results in this chapter focuses on resources available to and used by CBOs; the second section focuses on the resulting impacts. This chapter does not present all findings. Rather, it highlights key findings and cross-cutting issues arising from those findings. The presentation and discussion is based on the data and outcomes of the studies conducted as part of this evaluation as per the reports outlined in appendix A.

The potential for the community response to generate positive HIV and AIDS outcomes is real. Several reasons have been advanced to support this assertion. The four key arguments are the following:

- *Knowledge:* Communities (and the CBOs working with them) have greater knowledge about their HIV and AIDS-related needs.

- *Behavior:* Communities are best placed to engineer behavioral changes, as individual behaviors are often influenced by the social customs and norms of communities.
- *Capacity:* Communities (and community groups) have some basic capacity to identify, implement, and manage some HIV and AIDS activities. When activities are carried out by communities, there is more ownership, costs can be lower, and capacity is built within the community. This in turn strengthens long-term sustainability.
- *Social change:* The community response can strengthen social capital (in the form of increased trust and reduced stigma) through community mobilization. Likewise, it can also engineer positive social changes.

In addition, communities have the advantage of immediacy and locality—whereas it may take time for international organizations to roll out an effective response to local disease epidemics, the community is naturally on the front line of the response. Despite these advantages, the community response faces a number of challenges that can reduce its effectiveness:

- *Weak capacity:* The community response may be slower in expanding activities as communities may not have the necessary resources. There may also be significant costs in building the capacity of CBOs to manage activities and monitor results.
- *Accountability challenge:* Communities (and community groups) may lack the needed institutional framework to ensure that funds are used as intended, and they may face challenges in interacting with other partners. Community groups also face a risk that the availability of funding may induce a change in their activities such that they can no longer meet broader needs of their communities.
- *Funding challenge:* In many countries, CBOs are required to finance a counterpart share (if not all) of the recurrent costs (such as staff salaries) associated with the delivery of services. This may result in the extensive use of volunteers. The ability of many communities and CBOs to finance such costs can be quite limited. Donors and governments may need to consider supporting CBO recurrent costs under certain conditions (e.g., conditional cash transfers, results-based financing, or funds to fill the need for skilled personnel).

These facets of the community response are not specific to HIV and AIDS activities. However, they have become much more important in this context than in other fields due to the amount of resources that have been made available by the donor community. Have these resources generated concrete results? To answer this question, this evaluation analyzed whether the community response would generate the following:

- Increased knowledge about HIV and AIDS
- A reduction in risk behaviors
- Greater access to and utilization of HIV and AIDS services

- Significant differences in social transformation as demonstrated in improved gender relations, reduced stigmatization of those infected with and/or affected by HIV, and enhanced social cohesion
- Better HIV and health-related outcomes

The community response, which includes community caregivers, plays a unique role relative to other potential service providers who work in the community, but are not of the community. In many instances, CBOs show results in the most difficult circumstances, either political, geographical, or with regard to specific population groups. Some of the findings that will be discussed below are impressive precisely because CBOs/NGOs achieve results and affect the epidemic in the absence of a strong government response. At other times, the community response reaches populations or locations that are underserved. This also shows what a critical role communities and CBOs can play. Moreover, this role does not necessarily diminish simply because there is more government or international support in responding to HIV/AIDs. Rather, the role of the community response might shift due to a variety of influences. However, it would remain relevant to the extent that it continues to respond to the needs of communities. In this sense, communities are vital partners in the global approach to improving the effects and efficiencies of investments in HIV, AIDS, and health. The findings that follow cover both the inputs into community response and the outputs it produces. The first section focuses on what resources the community response has to draw on and how it utilizes these resources: roughly, the *size* of the response. The second section reports what effects have resulted—the *impact* of the response—and under what conditions.

Findings: Resources Available at the Community Level

Communities became much more involved in HIV and AIDS during the first decade of the twenty-first century than previously, and the number of community organizations providing HIV and AIDS services has increased significantly. Findings from this evaluation point to a number of factors underlying this growth. First is the nature of the epidemic itself. In Kenya, for instance, a large number of the surveyed CBOs indicated that they were created in response to the growing number of AIDS-related deaths in their communities. In Zimbabwe, the impact of increasing mortality and morbidity rates motivated existing grassroots organizations to have specific meetings dedicated to discussing HIV and AIDS.

The rapid increase in donor funding during the past decade is another factor motivating community engagement. Analysis of a sample of 349 civil society organizations in six southern African studies showed that the average level of spending on HIV and AIDS was almost three times higher in 2005 than in 2001 (Birdsall and Kelly 2007). Since then, further increases have taken place. Globally, the four major donors—Department for International Development (DfID), the Global Fund, President's Emergency Plan for AIDS Relief (PEPFAR), and the

World Bank—disbursed about US$690 million per year on average through civil society organizations (CSOs) during the 2003–09 period (Bonnel et al. 2011).[1] As shown by the analysis of CBO budgets in Kenya and Nigeria, donor funding for HIV and AIDS is reaching small CBOs. Financial assistance provided by bilateral and multilateral donors represented 33 percent of CBO budgets in Nigeria and 46 percent in Kenya (Kenya Evaluation Report 2011; Kenya HBCT Evaluation Report 2012; Nigeria Evaluation Report 2011).

Information on the activities of small NGOs and CBOs also came from a worldwide survey that was carried out in 2010 as part of this evaluation.[2] The 146 organizations that responded to the survey reported an allocation of expenditures that was markedly different from that of national HIV and AIDS programs. The largest share of expenditure was for prevention (42 percent). Within that category, expenditures were the largest for high-risk groups, reflecting the comparative advantage that NGOs/CBOs have in reaching such groups. This survey included all of the world's regions, not only Africa.

In contrast to national programs, the surveyed organizations indicated that they spent only 15 percent on treatment, mainly for supporting people living with HIV and AIDS (PLWHA). Nearly 19 percent was spent on care and support and on activities aimed at improving the enabling environment. The rest (6 percent) funded impact mitigation activities (see figure 3.1).

The analysis of flow of funds data from Kenya, Nigeria, and Zimbabwe revealed a somewhat different picture for these southern African countries (Katietek 2012).[3] Across the three countries, CBOs/NGOs reported spending the highest proportion of their funds on programs and activities related to support and mitigation of the economic impact of AIDS (27 percent), followed by treatment and care (20 percent), capacity building (16 percent), and finally

Figure 3.1 CBO/NGO Expenditures by Activities
percentage

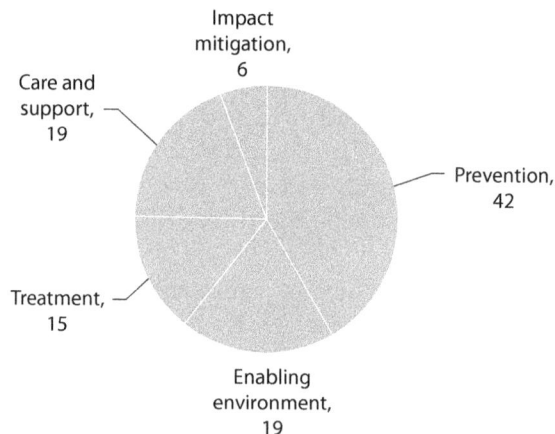

Source: International HIV/AIDS Alliance 2010 Survey in Bonnel et al. 2011.
Note: Percentages add up to 101 percent because of rounding.

program management (13 percent). The much larger proportion of funding allocated to support and mitigation reflected the more severe impact of the HIV epidemic in southern Africa.

How much of available resources flow to communities and how these resources are being used to fund countries' HIV response is of great interest to donors and governments. Yet relatively little is known about the magnitude of these resource flows to the community level. To address this knowledge gap, this evaluation conducted studies to (a) obtain a better understanding of donor-funding mechanisms and available donor funding at the country level available for the community response; (b) estimate the resources available to CBOs at the community level (as part of the evaluations in Kenya, Nigeria, and Zimbabwe); and (c) analyze in detail the budget of a few NGOs/CBOs. These analyses helped report the following characteristics:

- *The funding provided to civil society at the country level has become substantial.* In total, the four donors most actively involved in the AIDS response—PEPFAR, the Global Fund, the World Bank, and DfID[4]—have provided, on average, at least US$690 million a year during the 2003–2009 period. Part of this funding "directly" reached CSOs—meaning large and small national and international organizations. In addition, CSOs also received international funding through national channels. If this "indirect" funding is taken into account, it is likely that the total funding available for the community response would be higher (Bonnel et al. 2011).[5]

- *Donor funding is not reaching all organizations equally.* At the national level, most of the funds are disbursed to a few large international and national NGOs. This reflects the initial focus of the global AIDS response on achieving results quickly and in a manner that would meet the reporting requirement of donors.

- *National funding channels have become important for small NGOs and CBOs.* National commitments to build the community response facilitated the funding of a large number of small organizations and gave small NGOs and CBOs access to funding disbursed through national channels, including national NGO networks. In Kenya and Nigeria, for example, the surveyed CBOs indicated that national funding channels, mostly through the National AIDS Commission and their own fundraising, accounted for 55 and 67 percent of their expenditures, respectively (see figure 3.2).

- *Communities with a stronger response are able to mobilize more resources than communities with a weaker response.*[6] In Kenya, CBOs in communities with a stronger civil society engagement mobilized nearly three times more resources (US$21,400 versus US$7,500) and 40 percent more volunteers (24 versus 17) than CBOs located in communities with a weaker community response. In Nigeria, financial resources of CBOs in communities with strong civil society engagement were over three times larger (US$22,500 versus US$6,200) and

Figure 3.2 Funding Channels Mobilized by CBOs

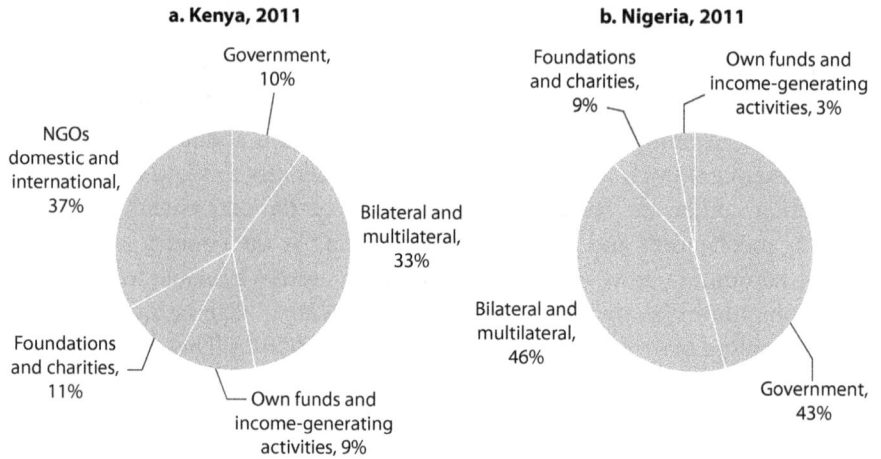

a. Kenya, 2011

Government, 10%

NGOs domestic and international, 37%

Bilateral and multilateral, 33%

Foundations and charities, 11%

Own funds and income-generating activities, 9%

b. Nigeria, 2011

Foundations and charities, 9%

Own funds and income-generating activities, 3%

Bilateral and multilateral, 46%

Government, 43%

Sources: Kenya Evaluation Report 2011; Nigeria Evaluation Report 2011.
Note: CBO = community-based organization, NGO = nongovernmental organization.

volunteers were 80 percent more numerous than in communities with a weaker community response.[7]

- *Volunteers are a crucial resource for CBOs.* Assigning a value to the unpaid labor of volunteers equal to the average compensation received by paid volunteers indicates that these resources amount to a large share of CBO financial resources: 40 percent in Kenya and 68 percent in Nigeria. On average, organizations with greater financial resources were able to employ more resources, suggesting that community groups are able to substantially leverage the mobilized financial resources (see box 3.1). However, the substantial role of volunteers introduces equity concerns as to whether these unpaid caregivers are carrying an undue burden in the community response.

- *The importance of volunteers for CBOs suggests that these organizations are more sustainable over the long term* than can be deduced by the high share of external resources in their funding. While the contributions of volunteers allow these CBOs to achieve more than could be expected, their high dependence on external resources is a cause for concern in a context of increased scarcity and calls to demonstrate efficiencies.

In conclusion, the funding amounts reaching the community, and thus CBOs, are smaller than originally expected. However, CBOs are capable of achieving results because of their own fundraising activities, in-kind contributions, use of volunteers, and the relatively small size of their catchment areas.

Box 3.1 The Role and Importance of Volunteers in Kenya, Nigeria, and Zimbabwe

Key findings:

- On average, CBOs employed 21 volunteers in Kenya and 36 in Nigeria; NGOs employed 205 volunteers per NGO.
- The majority of these organizations (63.3 percent) provided compensation, either in kind or in cash, to their volunteers.
- On average, volunteers worked 12 hours a week.
- Volunteers are a key resource. Assigning a monetary value to unpaid volunteer labor shows that these volunteers contribute an additional 46 percent to the financial resources of CBOs and NGOs in Zimbabwe.
- Volunteers in organizations that offered compensation worked fewer hours than unpaid volunteers but served a greater number of clients.

Source: Katietek 2012.

Findings: Effects of the Community Response

This section discusses the key findings of the evaluation of the community response to HIV and AIDS. A more detailed discussion of findings by country is presented in chapter 4, and summarized in table 3.1. The mixed-method approach to this evaluation means that the evidence has different degrees of robustness. In the last column of table 3.1, information is provided on the strength of the evidence for each of the main findings. See also box 3.2 for a classification of the levels of evidence. The source of the evidence shown in table 3.1 is the data presented in the studies and conducted for this evaluation (see appendix A).

Findings: Impact on Knowledge

Since the discovery of the HIV virus, nearly all countries have used some form of mass communication to increase knowledge. Recent evidence suggests that the effects of mass media are mixed and weak (Bertrand et al. 2006; Kaiser Family Foundation 2011) and may depend on their intensity, duration, number of messages, and outreach. Mass media messages have been shown to produce a dose-response effect, with greater exposure to messages increasing the likelihood of behavioral changes (Chomba et al. 2008). Consistent with previous findings, this evaluation revealed a mixed picture.

Prevention activities by CBOs revealed a mixed picture. Community-level activities such as theater plays, discussion with peer educators, television plays, and radio debates improved knowledge in Burkina Faso, but only in a partial way (Burkina Faso Evaluation Report 2011). Men and women retained knowledge differently and, unexpectedly, tolerance toward infected persons worsened (although the effect was small).

Table 3.1 Highlights of Evidence Concerning the Effects of the Community Response

Activities	Effects	General population	High-risk groups	Strength of evidence
Knowledge				
Information, awareness creation (speaking at public meetings, community theater, and so on)	Increased knowledge about HIV and AIDS	Burkina Faso Kenya Nigeria		Mixed evidence (+/-) Strong associative evidence Not statistically significant
Behaviors				
Promoting use of condoms	Increased condom use	Kenya Nigeria	India	Strong associative evidence Not statistically significant
Peer mentoring for HCT	Increased testing of HIV+ partner	Senegal		Causal evidence
Community group membership	Reduced risk behaviors	Zimbabwe	India	Strong associative evidence
Services				
HIV counseling and testing				
Peer mentoring for HCT	Increased testing and pick up	Senegal		Causal evidence
Group membership (women)	Increased testing	Zimbabwe		Strong associative evidence
Promotion of HCT, mobile HCT	Increased testing	Kenya, Nigeria		Not statistically significant
Home-based HCT	Increased testing	Kenya		Causal evidence
Empowerment of FSWs and MSM	Increased testing		India	Strong associative evidence
Prevention of mother-to-child transmission				
Provision of PMTCT services	Increased use	Zimbabwe		Strong associative evidence
Prevention services and care	Increased use	Nigeria (rural areas)		Strong suggestive evidence
Antiretroviral treatment				
Peer support adherence and nutrition	Increased timeliness of clinic and hospital visits	South Africa		Causal evidence

table continues next page

Table 3.1 Highlights of Evidence Concerning the Effects of the Community Response (continued)

Activities	Effects	General population	High-risk groups	Strength of evidence
Care and support				
Awareness of OVC rights	Increased awareness	Kenya		Strong suggestive evidence
Provision of support to OVC	Increased services (rural areas)	Nigeria		Strong suggestive evidence
Community group membership	Increased home-based care	Zimbabwe		Strong associative evidence
Mitigation of HIV effect				
Income-generating activities and material support for PLWHA	Increased PLWHA support	Kenya, Nigeria		Not statistically significant
Social change/transformation				
Stigma	Reduced/increased	Burkina Faso, Kenya, Lesotho, Nigeria, Zimbabwe		Mixed evidence
Gender rights, violence	Reduced police violence	Kenya, Nigeria	India	Mixed evidence
Empowerment of groups at high risk of infection	Increased access/use of social rights		India	Strong associative evidence
AIDS-Health Related Outcomes HIV and AIDS outcomes				
Community group membership	Reduced HIV incidence	Zimbabwe		Strong associative evidence
Empowerment of FSW groups	Lower STI		India	Strong associative evidence
Empowerment of MSM/Transgender	Lower STI		India	Not statistically significant

Sources: Burkina Faso Evaluation Report 2011; India Evaluation Report 2011; 2012a, 2012b; Kenya Evaluation Report 2011; Kenya HBCT Evaluation Report 2012; Lesotho Evaluation Report 2011; Nigeria Evaluation Report 2011; Senegal Evaluation Report 2010; South Africa Evaluation Report 2011; Zimbabwe Evaluation Report 2011a, 2011b, 2012.

Note: AIDS = acquired immune deficiency syndrome, ART = antiretroviral therapy, FSW = female sex worker, HCT = HIV counseling and testing, HBCT = home-based counseling and testing, HIV = human immunodeficiency virus, MSM = men who have sex with men, OVC = orphans and vulnerable children, PLWHA = people living with HIV and AIDS, PMTCT = prevention of mother-to-child transmission, STI = sexually transmitted infection.

Box 3.2 Classification of the Strength of the Evidence

- *Strong causal evidence*: This rating was applied to evaluations that are able to prove the existence of a causal relationship between a program and its results (randomized control trial, or RCT).
- *Strong associative evidence:* A slightly lower level of evidence is obtained when the same association between an intervention and its outcome is found through a prospective cohort study. A similar rating was given when quasi-experimental evaluations showed associations that were corroborated by other evaluation studies.
- *Strong suggestive evidence:* This rating was given when a statistically significant association between a program and an output was found in only one country or in one variation of an indicator. It implies that additional evaluations may be needed to confirm this finding.
- *Mixed evidence:* This characterizes results that are contradicted by another evaluation's findings. This rating also applies when evidence varies on the same indicators (e.g., stigma) between positive and negative effects.

However, there is evidence that systematic and targeted community-level activities can increase knowledge. In Kenya's Western and Nyanza provinces that were one of the foci of this evaluation, all of the surveyed CBOs indicated that information and education activities had been implemented. These included delivering systematic outreach programs targeted to various population groups and public meeting places. Invariably, CBOs mentioned increasing the level of awareness and knowledge as their main achievement. This was confirmed by the evaluation's results (Kenya Evaluation Report 2011). Community members in communities with a strong CBO presence had almost 15 times higher odds than respondents in the comparison group of knowing that using a condom reduces the chance of becoming infected with HIV (aOR = 14.67; 95 percent CI = 7.73–27.85) (see figure 3.3).

However, CBOs' general advocacy and dissemination of knowledge about HIV is unlikely to have a measurable impact when knowledge is already high. In Nigeria, existing knowledge was already high,[8] and other sources of information had already reached communities: 94 percent of the surveyed households indicated that they had seen or heard messages about HIV through various media such as the radio. Not surprisingly, there was no indication that CBO activities affected knowledge.

Thus, the key finding is that community responses can increase HIV and AIDS-related knowledge. This is more likely to happen when communities and CBOs engage in systematic and targeted community-level activities with clear expectations as to the purpose of increasing knowledge (e.g., which behaviors are targeted). The traditional approach to broad informational

Figure 3.3 Associations between Strength of CBO Engagement and HIV Knowledge
Kenya 2011

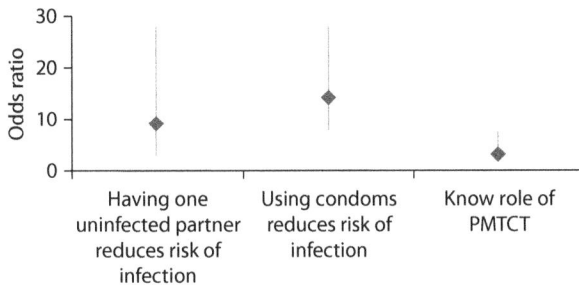

Source: Kenya Evaluation Report 2011.
Note: Square = adjusted odds ratio, Line = 95 percent confidence interval, PMTCT = prevention of mother-to-child transmission.

types of activities was perhaps needed more in the earlier period of the epidemic. Now, as general knowledge of HIV and AIDS is more widespread, targeted interventions are more likely to achieve results, whether to introduce a new program, scale up an existing one, or generate demand for specific services.

Findings: From Knowledge to Risk Reduction

Standard behavioral interventions are often based on models of cognitive behavior that assume that people will change their behaviors if they are fully informed. Yet there are many examples of countries where, despite high knowledge about HIV, little behavioral change has taken place. In such contexts, empowerment, strong community mobilization, and involvement in community groups may provide the levers for changing the norms and social values that influence individual behavior.

There is strong associative evidence that empowerment of groups at high risk of infections, such as female sex workers (FSWs) and men who have sex with men (MSM), can lead to behavioral changes (India Evaluation Report 2011, 2012b). Developing a framework for measuring the empowerment process and evaluating its impact was the focus of two studies carried out for this evaluation in Karnataka state and Andhra Pradesh state in India. Although both studies developed slightly different frameworks to report and measure empowerment, the results were similar: empowerment was associated with positive behavioral changes, especially in terms of increased condom use. One dimension of empowerment (*power within*, which measured self-esteem, motivation, and confidence) was strongly associated with condom use among FSWs in Karnataka state (see table 3.2).

The intensity of community mobilization matters. Strong empowerment of FSWs and Men who have sex with men and transgender individuals (MSM/Ts) measured by collectivization was associated with higher consistent condom use with occasional and regular clients[9] (occasional clients: aOR = 1.8, 95 percent

Table 3.2 Association between Empowerment and HIV Risk among Female Sex Workers (FSW), Adjusted for Background Characteristics among All Districts (Karnataka State, India, 2010)[a]

	Power within	Power with	Power over
Condom use at last sex with occasional client	0.03	0.166	0.46
Frequency of condom use with occasional client	0.02	0.62***	−0.15
Condom use at last sex with regular client	−0.08	0.65***	0.49**
Frequency of condom use with regular client	−0.04	0.67***	−0.18
Condom use at last sex with regular partner	0.03	0.16*	0.07
Frequency of condom use at last sex with regular partner	0.15	0.18*	0.07

Source: India Evaluation Report 2011.

Note: B values are obtained from a binary logistic regression. *p* values are summarized as follows: *$p < .05$; **$p < .01$; ***$p < .001$.
a. The empowerment process of community groups of FSWs in Karnataka State was measured by three indicators: *power within* was created from variables that measured self-esteem, motivation, and confidence. *Power with* was defined to measure the respondent's confidence in the ability of sex workers to work together for various purposes. *Power over* measured social rights, such as ownership of a ration card or having a bank account.

CI: 1.2–2.6; regular clients: aOR = 1.7, 95 percent CI: 1.2–2.4) (India Evaluation Report 2012b) (see figure 3.4). Similar effects were found among MSM/T. One dimension of empowerment—high collective efficacy—was significantly associated with higher consistent use of condoms with paying partners (aOR = 1.9; 95 percent CI = 1.5–2.3).[10]

Participation in community groups and frequent discussion of HIV- and AIDS-related issues are two important characteristics of effective community activities. Indeed, the evaluation in Zimbabwe indicated that community group membership can have strong protective effects, provided that (a) groups actively and frequently discuss HIV and AIDS-related issues, and (b) there is strong interpersonal communication about AIDS-related deaths or experiences (Zimbabwe Evaluation Report 2011a, 2011b, 2012).

Analysis of community groups in the region of Matabeland, Zimbabwe, revealed extensive participation in community groups (43 percent of women at baseline in 1998), with frequent discussion of HIV-related issues within these groups (over 60 percent of community groups discussed HIV issues between 1998 and 2003). Information sharing about HIV was catalyzed by a communication process that relied on interpersonal communication and exchange of information through social networks, a process that has been viewed as one of the factors behind Ugandan population behavioral changes (Low-Beer and Stoneburger 2004). These processes provided a pathway linking community group membership and improved health outcomes (see box 3.3).

However, the protective effects of group membership are not automatically guaranteed. Effects in Zimbabwe, for instance, differed across groups, between men and women, and over time: group participation was more effective in the earlier stage of the epidemic (1998–2003) than later during the years 2003–08. Figure 3.5 shows that women who participate in community groups are significantly more likely to reduce their risk behavior, whereas for men the impact is much smaller.

Figure 3.4 Effects of Low and High Collectivization among FSW on Condom Use

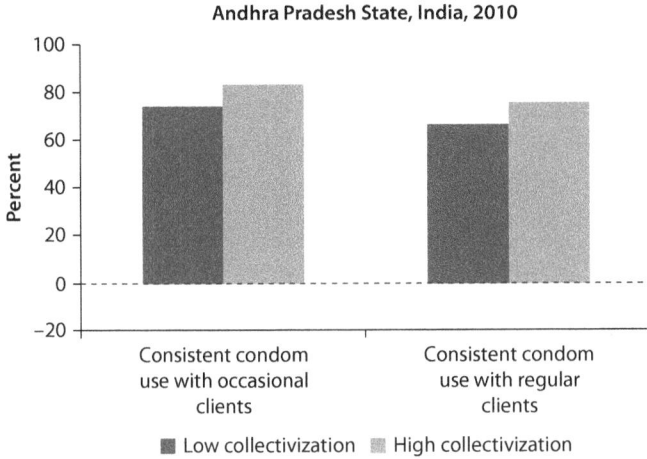

Andhra Pradesh State, India, 2010

Source: India Evaluation Report 2012b.

Box 3.3 What Are the Pathways between Community Group Membership and Health?

Purposeful dialogue in community groups often results in the following:

- Sharing of vital information about HIV
- Translation of medical information into locally appropriate concepts and new behavioral norms
- A sense of confidence to implement the new norms
- A sense of urgency and motivation to respond effectively to HIV through the sharing of emotionally charged personal experiences
- A sense of common purpose around the need for individuals to make the best of services, and for people to assist the AIDS-affected wherever possible
- Sharing of information about other sources of support

All of these factors potentially result in less risky behavior, a culture of solidarity, and mutual support and better use of prevention, treatment, care, and support. Participation in community groups enables members to engage in critical dialogue about HIV and AIDS.

Source: Zimbabwe Evaluation Report 2012.

The effects of the community response on behaviors are weaker in Burkina Faso, Kenya, and Nigeria. These countries have much lower HIV prevalence and geographically mixed epidemics (concentrated with high HIV prevalence in some areas, and generalized with much lower HIV prevalence in others). In Kenya, there was a strong association between the strength of CBO engagement and condom use: respondents in high CBO-engagement communities had four times higher odds of reporting consistent condom use with all sex partners in

Figure 3.5 Community Groups and Low-Risk Behavior in Zimbabwe (1998–2003)

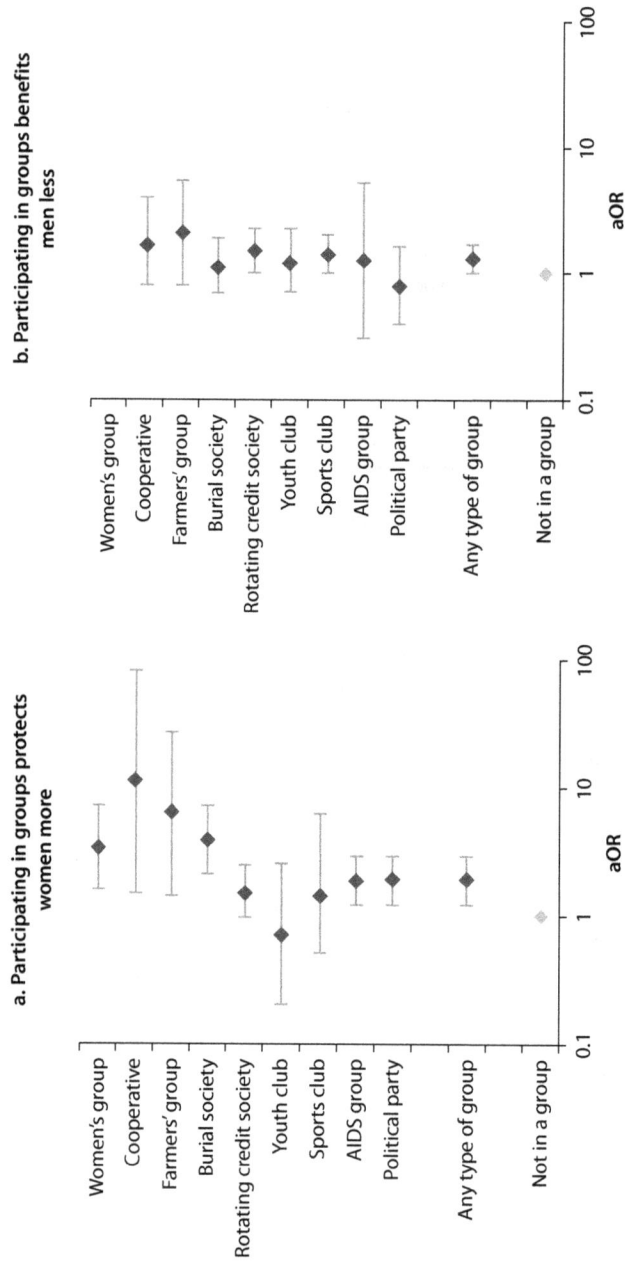

a. Participating in groups protects women more

b. Participating in groups benefits men less

Source: Gregson et al. 2011. Reprinted with permission from the Population Council.
Note: Risk reduction was defined either as a reduction in the number of new sexual partners in the past year or continuing to report one or no new partners in the year before the survey, as these were the main factors behind Zimbabwe's decline in HIV prevalence. Diamond = age-adjusted odds ratio (aOR), 95 percent confidence interval; 1=no change; 1–100 increases in odds of reducing risk behaviors.

the previous 12 months (OR: 4.09, 95 percent CI: 2.30–7.27) than respondents in comparison communities. There were no other visible associations with other measures of sexual behavior.

Similarly, in Burkina Faso, the study found that greater prevention activities at the village level were associated with an increase in the use of condoms with a second partner, but not with other changes in sexual behaviors (Burkina Faso Evaluation Report 2011). In Nigeria, the evaluation found no relationship between the strength of CBO engagement and any measures of sexual risk behavior (condom use and numbers of sex partners).

A poor match between needs and CBO activities contributes to lower impact. In Nigeria, for instance, over half of the surveyed CBOs indicated that they carried out information and education campaigns (IEC), but only 3 percent of the interviewed CBOs reported engaging in behavioral change communication. Furthermore, there were significant shortcomings in the use and distribution of condoms. Only 23 percent of the survey respondents who had more than one sex partner in the last year reported consistent condom use. However, only 20 percent of CBOs in the study communities and 28 percent of CBOs in the comparison communities indicated that they were involved in condom social marketing. Although in the past IEC was relevant in increasing HIV knowledge, it is no longer the best intervention to achieve behavioral change leading to greater condom use. Other, more specific, and better targeted interventions are needed, whether social marketing or purposeful community dialogue. Thus, given the IEC focus of CBOs in Nigeria, it was not surprising to find little effect of community activities on behavioral change.

In conclusion, the *intensity* of community mobilization matters for its impact on behavior. Participation in community groups and frequent discussion of HIV- and AIDS-related issues are two important characteristics of effective community activities. They empower groups at high risk of infections, such as FSWs and MSM, which can, in turn, lead to behavioral changes. However, the protective effects of group membership are not automatically guaranteed. The groups need to be purposeful.

It should be noted, however, that the effects of the community response on behaviors are weaker in Burkina Faso, Kenya, and Nigeria than elsewhere in this evaluation. One possible explanation is that in these countries there seems to be a poor match between community needs and CBO activities, which contributes to the lack of apparent results.

Findings: Community Mobilization and the Use of HIV- and AIDS-Related Services

A crucial step on the pathway from community intervention to impact on health-related outcomes is ensuring access to and utilization of services. Although the community response is unlikely to have much effect on the availability of services—with the exception of home-based care, support for PLWHA and orphaned and vulnerable children (OVC), and mitigation—it has the potential to increase the use of such services. This is more likely to take place when the impact of the HIV epidemic is severe in the community and on caregivers[11] when there is dedicated support from community members, and when there is a strong referral system in place.

The community response can increase the demand for health services in the context of a concentrated HIV epidemic among groups at high risk of infection. This is especially the case when the prevalence of HIV and sexually transmitted infections (STIs) is already high among FSWs and when the legal environment is not overly repressive. In this context, community empowerment can increase the use of health facilities. This was observed among FSWs in the Andhra Pradesh state of India. The proportion of FSWs who reported visiting a government health facility for STI treatment was significantly higher among those with a medium level of collectivization as compared to those with a low level of collectivization (60.4 versus 42.2 percent, aOR = 2.1, 95 percent CI:1.3–3.2) (India Evaluation Report 2012b).[12]

Addressing the issue of stigma and a repressive environment remains a major hurdle to increasing MSM's use of health services. Stigma still represents a significant barrier to service uptake, as shown by the studies in India and Burkina Faso. For instance, the Karnataka state study provided no evidence that MSM/T empowerment increased the use of health facilities. One reason is the perception by MSM/Ts of the stigma that is prevalent among health providers toward this population. This suggests that there is a need to develop innovative strategies to break the barriers that prevent MSM/Ts from accessing health services. Furthermore, there is a need to raise awareness among MSM/Ts about STIs that are often asymptomatic. Hence, there is urgency for this population to access and use health services.

Community response can increase the demand for services (strong associative evidence). Participation in community groups can stimulate the exchange of information about health services and induce group members to seek specific health services. This effect was noticeable among women in Zimbabwe: 41 percent of women in community groups versus 30 percent of women not in groups had taken HIV counseling and testing (HCT) between 2003 and 2008 (aOR = 1.5, 95 percent CI:1.2–1.8). Other positive effects included increased uptake of PMTCT by women (51.7 versus 35.7 percent; aOR = 1.7, CI:1.2–2.6), and greater provision of care by women (45 versus 30 percent) during the period 2003–08 (Zimbabwe Evaluation Report 2012).

A similar effect was observed in Nigeria. CBOs were involved in providing a variety of treatment (antiretroviral treatment and treatment of opportunistic infections); care (home-based care and home visits); and support (financial, material and psychological support). However, the effects of CBO engagement were most noticeable in rural areas: an increase of one in the number of CBOs per 100,000 people was associated with a twofold increase in the odds that a respondent would report using prevention services in rural areas, and a 64 percent increase in the odds of reporting treatment access (see figure 3.6).

Although this evaluation did not find statistically significant results related to OVC in Nigeria or in Kenya, a systematic review of the existing OVC literature

Figure 3.6 CBO Density and Service Use (Odds of Utilization)

Nigeria, Rural Areas, 2011

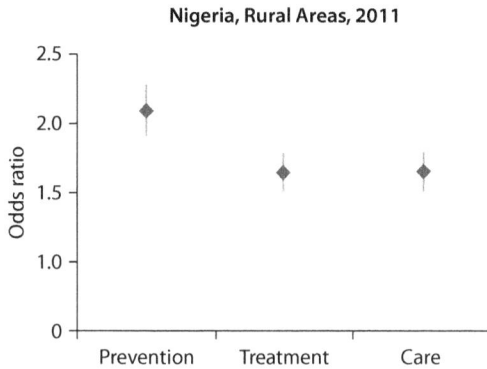

Source: Nigeria Evaluation Report 2011.
Note: Diamonds = adjusted odds ratio, vertical line = 95 percent confidence interval.

on the effects of the community response to HIV and AIDS on "child outcomes"—specifically evaluating community-based interventions—found that communities were playing a role in delivering, hosting, facilitating, and providing key elements of the HIV response, including the response to OVC. Of the studies reviewed, 86 percent showed positive child outcomes (Sherr 2010).[13]

Broad community member and leader involvement can increase the demand for services and overcome the adverse effects of stigma (causal relation). In Kenya, the evaluation of a community-wide, home-based counseling and testing (HBCT) campaign found that large-scale HIV testing can be implemented successfully in the presence of stigma, most likely because of its "whole community approach" (Kenya HBCT Evaluation Report 2012). By avoiding the need for individuals to single themselves out to seek testing, HBCT can blunt the impact of stigma on testing uptake. As a result, HBCT increased the probability of being tested for HIV by about 70 percent for individuals who were initially living in one of the treatment locations. Furthermore, HBCT reached people who had never before had an HIV test: the percentage of people who have ever received an HIV test rose from 64 percent in the control groups to 95 percent in the treatment areas, a 31 percentage point gain.

Dedicated support from community peer members is effective (causal evidence). This was found in the case of both peer mentoring for HTC in Senegal and peer adherence support for antiretroviral treatment in South Africa.

In Senegal, the evaluation found strong causal evidence that, when compared to unfunded traditional social mobilization activities,[14] peer mentoring doubled the number of individuals attending pre-HIV test counseling and those being tested. Mentoring also increased the number of individuals receiving their test results—by about 120 percent ($p < .1$) (Senegal Evaluation Report 2010) (see figure 3.7). In addition, peer mentoring was effective in changing the behavior of individuals who test positive. The number of HIV-positive individuals whose

Figure 3.7 Peer Mentoring Compared to Unfunded Traditional Sensitization Activities
percentage increase in numbers

Senegal, 2010

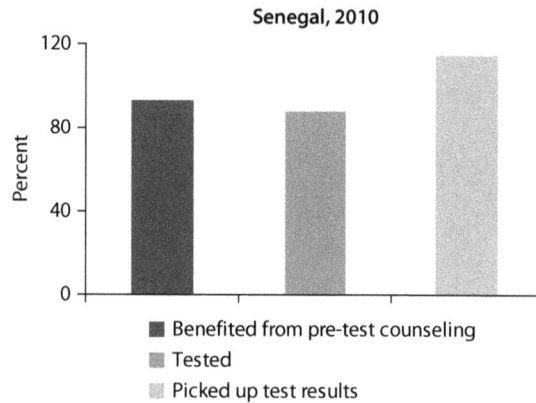

■ Benefited from pre-test counseling
▨ Tested
▨ Picked up test results

Source: Senegal Evaluation Report 2010.

partners were tested ($p < .1$) rose by about 60 percent compared to traditional sensitization activities.

Peer adherence support combined with nutrition can increase the timeliness of scheduled hospital visits for antiretroviral treatment. Antiretroviral therapy (ART) clients who were visited twice weekly at their homes by a peer adherence supporter had statistically significant lower delays in scheduled clinic visits than those who did not receive such peer support (-15.8 days; p < .05; 95 percent CI -29.1: -2.4) (South Africa Evaluation Report 2011). Delays in scheduled hospital visits were lower only for those receiving both adherence and nutritional support (-32.5 days; p < .01; 95 percent CI: -56.7 to -8.4). These findings represent strong causal evidence that peer support improves the timeliness of adult clinic and hospital visits. However, the evaluation failed to find evidence that peer support had a significant impact on self-reported measures of adherence.[15]

What was learned is that the community response can increase the demand for take-up of health services in the context of generalized and concentrated HIV epidemics among groups at high risk of infection. Dedicated support from community members, such as peer mentoring, appears more effective than less-personalized approaches. However, stigma and a repressive environment remain major hurdles to increasing the use of HIV and AIDS services in general, and to increasing access to health services by the most at-risk populations such as FSWs and MSM/Ts. Encouragingly, broad involvement of community members and leaders may be able to overcome stigma's discouraging impact by ensuring that no individual is singled out. Organized groups such as home-based care alliances and caregivers for AIDS networks are more important than ever as agents of community development and service delivery and can provide a bridge between the facility-based care and communities.

Findings: Community Response and Social Changes

Communities have now become a crucial component of HIV and AIDS strategies. For instance, the UNAIDS' "Five-pillar Treatment 2.0" states that "community-based approaches to build trust, protect human rights and provide opportunities for socialization directly improve the ability of people to use HIV services and to benefit from antiretroviral therapy and prevent new infections" (UNAIDS 2010). In this approach, social transformation is viewed as an important output of the community response.

The evidence from the country evaluations indicates that there are complex pathways that depend substantially on the population groups, country contexts, geographic location, and the overall government policy.

The community response can foster social changes among groups that are severely affected by the HIV epidemic. In India, the evaluation found a strong association between empowerment of FSWs and MSM/Ts and social change. Being a member of a sex worker community group was associated with access to social entitlements ($p < .05$); reduced violence ($p < .001$); and reduced police coercion ($p < .001$) (India Evaluation Report 2012a). Among Zimbabwe's general population, the community response led to significant changes in sexual risk perception and a reduction in stigmatizing attitudes toward PLWHA: for women, 2.5 versus 5 percent (aOR = 0.6 CI: 0.3–1.0); for men 3.5 versus 9 percent (aOR = 0.4 CI:01–0.9) (Zimbabwe Evaluation Report 2011b).

However, the effects of community programs are gender sensitive, indicating the need to implement different types of programs to reach both men and women. Examples include the following: prevention programs in Burkina Faso's communities affected men's and women's differently as related to knowledge of HIV, awareness of ART and stigma towards the infected. In Senegal, peer mentoring had strong effects on men's HIV testing and counseling, while standard forms of community mobilization were more effective for women. In Zimbabwe, group membership was found to be more beneficial for women than for men.

The country's context and governmental policies toward commercial sex work and MSM can make great differences. In India, sex work is illegal, but it is not a criminal offence. This opened the door to a dialogue with the police, which resulted in reduced police violence. In contrast, stigma attached to MSM/Ts and the existence of a repressive environment generally prevented MSM/T from accessing health services.

Changes in gender norms and children's rights may more properly be the domain of national policymakers than community organizations. CBOs were not found to have a large impact on gender violence and norms, but changes at the national level such as laws and policies appear to have an impact at the local level. In Kenya, key informants perceived declines in violence against women as linked primarily to changes in national policies (such as the introduction of free primary-level education and the adoption of legislation protecting women from violence). In Nigeria, increased awareness, social consequences for the perpetrators, and the influence of government, NGOs, and other local organizations, were often cited as reasons for the decline. It is also possible that CBO activities at the community level heightened the perception of gender inequalities and influenced voting.

Outside factors may also have greater influence on children's rights than does CBO activity. Respondents in Kenya's study communities indicated that community members were about 25 percent more likely to be aware of institutions that promote and protect children's rights (aOR: 1.25, 95 percent CI: 1.62–7.46) in areas with high levels of community response. However, Nigeria's evaluation did not find any effect of the community response on children's rights. Key informants attributed changes on children's rights to other factors, such as national policies and increasing educational attainment (Kenya Evaluation Report 2011; Nigeria Evaluation Report 2011).

Community HIV and AIDS programs can have unintended adverse consequences on stigmatization, and should therefore be designed with this in mind. For instance, a negative, albeit small association was found between prevention programs and men's tolerance toward infected persons (5 percent confidence level) (Burkina Faso Evaluation Report 2011). This suggests that prevention programs could exacerbate personal stigmatizing attitudes by creating greater awareness of the disease. A similar consequence resulted from HBCT in Kenya. HBCT was found to lower the level of stigma of community leaders but to raise the communities' level of anger and disgust felt toward HIV-positive individuals (Kenya HBCT Evaluation Report 2012). These results indicate a need for redoubling efforts to deal squarely with stigma and discrimination. It is possible that communities and CBOs are ill equipped to address these deeply ingrained feelings in people. Qualitative approaches such as those based on community dialogue may prove helpful in changing community member beliefs and practices.

In conclusion, the community response can foster social changes among those most affected by the HIV epidemic. However, the effects of community-based activities are gender sensitive, suggesting the need to implement programs that are appropriate for reaching men or women. It is also important to be mindful of the potential unintended adverse consequences of certain activities. Finally, community responses cannot supplant the role of governmental policies, which can have a large influence on norms surrounding everything from MSM to domestic abuse.

Findings: Community Response and HIV Health-Related Outcomes

One of the most desired impacts of community responses are those that show statistically significant biological outcomes. As the primary objective of any HIV program is the reduction of HIV infections, results that indicate a convincing impact of community responses on the number of HIV infections or other health outcomes are critical. This evaluation found this impact in two different epidemiological settings.

There is strong suggestive evidence that empowerment of FSWs and community group membership can improve biological outcomes. Analysis of two rounds of the Integrated Biological and Behavioral Assessment (IBBA) (4,699 FSWs) that was conducted in five districts of Karnataka State, India, between 2005 and 2009 indicated that community group membership compared to nonmembership was associated with lower prevalence of STIs, for example, chlamydia and gonorrhea (aOR = 0.95, $p < .001$) and active syphilis (aOR = 0.98, $p < .05$) (India Evaluation Report 2011). There was less evidence that community group membership affected HIV prevalence among FSWs. The HIV prevalence was lower among FSWs who were community group members, but the difference was not statistically significant. This may be in part a reflection of the composition of the group of FSWs. Most of the women in the survey had been sex workers for some time, and infection might have occurred earlier upon sex work initiation. This indicates that unless FSWs become members of an empowered group soon after they begin sex work, the social mobilization of FSWs may not translate rapidly into lower HIV prevalence among them. However, social mobilization would still protect the broader population as a result of the increased use of condoms. These effects are consistent with other studies, which have noted that among high-risk groups, high condom use has a demonstrable population-level effect.

Community group membership can lead to reduced HIV incidence depending on the severity and stage of the HIV epidemic. Zimbabwe is one of the few sub-Saharan African countries for which there is compelling evidence for sustained decline in HIV prevalence driven by reduced levels of risk behavior (Gregson et al. 2010) (see figure 3.8).[16] Halperin et al. (2011) attribute this decline to changes in sexual behavior as a result of personal observation of AIDS deaths and interpersonal communications that played a key role in transmitting information. Evidence from this evaluation suggests that group membership played an important role in the decline in national HIV prevalence. Strong associative evidence was found that participation in a community group was associated with reduced HIV incidence for women (aIRR = 0.64, CI: 0.43–0.94) during the period 1998–2003 (Zimbabwe Evaluation Report 2011b and Gregson et al. 2011). New findings from the Zimbabwe Evaluation Report indicate that for HIV incidence, (i) there was a dose effect in 1998–2003; and (ii) the effect of group membership disappeared in the subsequent period (2003–2008). In the later period (2003–08), the decline in HIV incidence may have slowed (Halperin et al. 2011), a trend consistent with the apparent lack of effects of the community response on HIV incidence.

The key lesson is that the community response can decrease HIV (and STI) incidence and prevalence under circumstances where the government response is limited. However, this effect is dependent on gender and setting.

Figure 3.8 Community Group Participation and HIV Incidence among Women and Men in Zimbabwe (1998–2003)

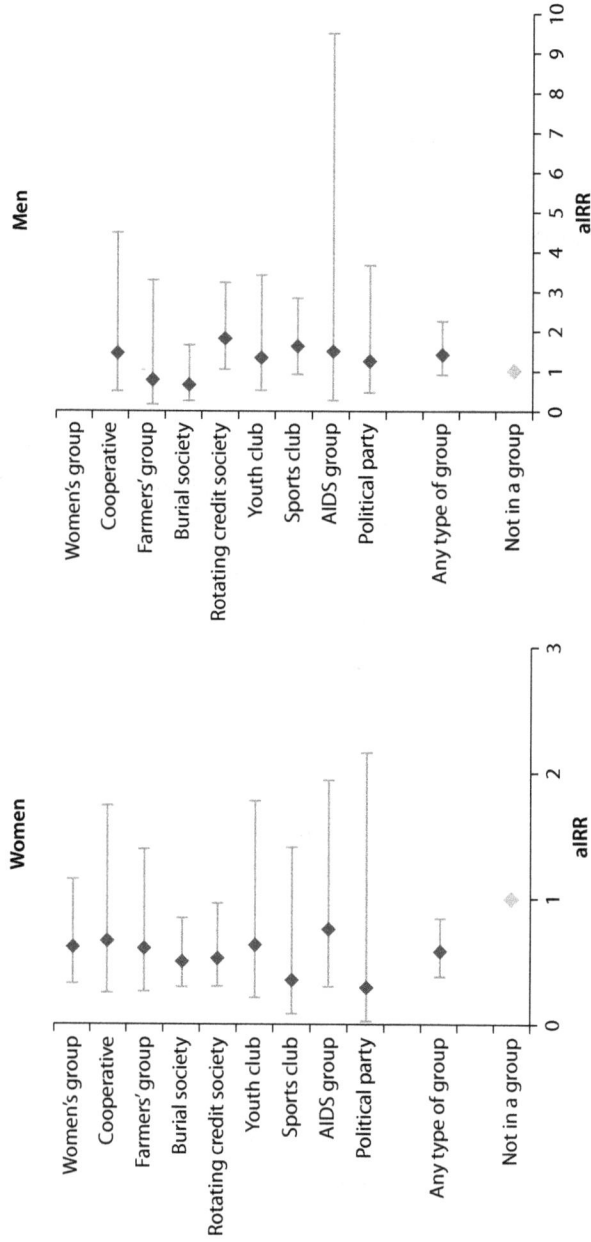

Source: Gregson et al. 2011. Reprinted with permission from the Population Council.
Note: Diamonds = age-adjusted incidence rate ratio (aIRR) and 95 percent confidence interval for HIV infection for individuals in community groups at baseline compared to those not in a group, by form of community group.

Notes

1. Due to data limitations, it was not possible to retrace the evolution over time of the funding for CSOs. However, it is likely to have risen in line with the global funding for the AIDS response.

2. These organizations were mainly small—two-thirds had fewer than 20 members—and they were mainly based in developing countries (89 percent) with a spread covering all regions.

3. The surveyed organizations were small CBOs in Kenya and Nigeria and medium-size CBOs/NGOs in Zimbabwe.

4. Together, these four donors account for more than 80 percent of the funding provided by donor governments to civil society (Kaiser Family Foundation 2011).

5. Information on the direct and indirect funding is not readily available from the donors' centralized database as donors do not routinely disaggregate funding by implementing partners (e.g., government, civil society, international organizations). In the case of the World Bank, it was estimated that the total funding (including both direct and indirect channels) provided to NGOs/CBOs amounted to 39 percent of World Bank funding for HIV and AIDS projects. The Global Fund estimates that about one third of their country expenditures at the end of the 2009 funding cycle went to CSOs and academia (Global Fund 2011).

6. The strength of the community response was measured by the number of CBOs in specific geographic areas in Kenya and by the number of CBOs per 100,000 people in Nigeria.

7. These estimates are based on the surveyed organizations. Due to the small sample size (56 in two of six states in Nigeria, 25 in two western provinces in Kenya, and 12 in the region of Matabeland in Zimbabwe), they are not necessarily representative at the national level.

8. For instance, 89 percent of the respondents knew that having one, uninfected partner reduces the chances of contracting HIV, and 79 percent knew that using a condom reduces the chances of contracting HIV.

9. Collectivization was measured among FSWs in terms of three binary (low, high) indices of collective efficacy, collective agency, and collective action. Collectivization among MSM/T was measured by participation in a public event and binary index (low, high) of collective efficacy.

10. "Collective efficacy" is the belief of the affected community in its power to work together. It is defined as the choice, control, and power that groups have to act to claim their rights (whether political, social, and/or economic). Collective action is represented by the organized activities that community members take to enact their agenda. For more, see India Evaluation Report (2011).

11. The UK Consortium on AIDS and International Development has differentiated between primary caregivers (lay persons) and secondary caregivers (community or other health workers) (UK Consortium 2012).

12. For FSWs, a summary measure of collectivization was computed based on the three distinct dimensions of collectivization (collective efficacy, collective agency, and collective action).

13. This study was commissioned for this evaluation. For more information about OVC, see UNICEF's Social Protection Strategic Framework and other publications, http://www.unicef.org/socialprotection/framework/index_61577.html.

14. Traditional unfunded sensitization programs are the activities that are carried out routinely at the community level without additional funding aimed at promoting counseling and testing.

15. This study conducted with and by the World Bank research group is still ongoing.

16. HIV prevalence peaked in Zimbabwe at 26.5 percent around 1997, before falling steadily to 14.3 percent in 2009.

References

Bertrand J. T., K. O'Reilly, J. Denison, R. Anhang, and M. Sweat. 2006. "Systematic Review of the Effectiveness of Mass Communication Programs to Change HIV/AIDS-Related Behaviors in Developing Countries." *Health Education Research* 21 (4): 567–97.

Birdsall, K., and K. Kelly. 2007. *Community Responses to HIV/AIDS in South Africa: Findings from a Multi-Community Study.* Johannesburg: Centre for AIDS Development, Research and Evaluation (CADRE).

Bonnel, R., R. Rodriguez-Garcia, J. Olivier, Q. Wodon, S. McPherson, K. Orr, and J. Ross. 2011. "Funding Mechanisms for the Community Response to HIV and AIDS." Background Paper, World Bank, Washington, DC.

Burkina Faso Evaluation Report. 2011. *Social and Individual Behaviour Change Initiated by Prevention Activities and Antiretroviral Treatment Provision in Burkina Faso.* Washington, DC: World Bank.*

Chomba, E., S. Allen, W. Kanweka, A. Tichacek, G. Cox, E. Shutes, I. Zulu, N. Kancheya, M. Sinkala, R. Stephenson, and A. Haworth; Rwanda Zambia HIV Research Group. 2008. "Evolution of Couples' Voluntary Counseling and Testing for HIV in Lusaka, Zambia." *Journal of Acquired Immune Deficiency Syndromes* 47 (1): 108–15.

Gregson, S., E. Gonese, T. B. Hallett, N. Taruberekera, J. W. Hargrove, E. L. Corbett, R. Dorrington, S. Dube, K. Dehne, and O. Mugurungi. 2010. "HIV Decline Due to Reductions in Risky Sex in Zimbabwe? Evidence from a Comprehensive Epidemiological Review." *International Journal of Epidemiology* 39 (5): 1311–23.

Gregson, S., P. Mushati, H. Grusin, M. Nhamo, C. Schumacher, et al. 2011. "Social Capital and Reduced Female Vulnerability to HIV Infection in Rural Zimbabwe." *Population and Development Review* 37: 333–59.

Global Fund. 2011. *Making a Difference Results Report.* Geneva: The Global Fund to Fight AIDS, Tuberculosis and Malaria.

Halperin, D. T., O. Mugurungi, T. B. Hallett, B. Muchini, B. Campbell, T. Magure, C. Benedikt, and S. Gregson. 2011. "A Surprising Prevention Success: Why Did the HIV Epidemic Decline in Zimbabwe?" *PLoS Medicine* 8 (2): e1000414.

India Evaluation Report. 2011. *Evaluation of Community Mobilization and Empowerment in Relation to HIV Prevention among Female Sex Workers in Karnataka State, South India.* Washington, DC: World Bank.*

———. 2012a. "Using Data to Understand Programmatic Shifts in the Avahan HIV Prevention Program at the Community Level." World Bank, Washington, DC.

———. 2012b. *Community Collectivization and Its Association with Selected Outcomes among Female Sex Workers and High-Risk Men Who Have Sex with Men/Transgenders in Andhra Pradesh, India.* Washington, DC: World Bank.*

Kaiser Family Foundation. 2011. *Global Health Interventions: A Review of Evidence.* Washington, DC: Kaiser Family Foundation. www.globalhealth.kff.org/GHIR.aspx.

Katietek, J. 2012. *Flow of Funds in Community-based Organizations in Kenya, Nigeria and Zimbabwe.* Study Report. World Bank, Washington, DC.

Kenya Evaluation Report. 2011. *Effects of the Community Response on HIV and AIDS in Kenya.* Washington, DC: World Bank.*

Kenya HBCT Evaluation Report. 2012. *The Links between Home-Based HIV Counseling and Testing and HIV Stigma in Western Kenya.* Washington, DC: World Bank.*

Lesotho Evaluation Report. 2011. "Combating the AIDS Pandemic in Lesotho by Understanding Beliefs and Behaviors." World Bank, Washington, DC.

Low-Beer, D., and R. Stoneburger. 2004. "AIDS Communications through Social Networks: Catalyst for Behaviour Changes in Uganda." *African Journal of AIDS Research* 3 (1): 1–13.

Nigeria Evaluation Report. 2011. *Effects of the Community Response to HIV and AIDS in Nigeria.* Washington, DC: World Bank.*

Senegal Evaluation Report. 2010. "HIV/AIDS Sensitization, Social Mobilization and Peer-Mentoring: Evidence from a Randomized Experiment." World Bank, Washington, DC.

Sherr, L. 2010. *Efficacy of Community-Based Organizational Input on Supporting Orphans and Vulnerable Children (OVC) Outcomes in Relation to HIV 2004–2009: OVC; A Systematic Review.* Background paper, World Bank, Washington, DC.

South Africa Evaluation Report. 2011. *Timely Peer Adherence and Nutritional Support in Free State Province's Public Sector Antiretroviral Treatment Program.* Washington, DC: World Bank.*

UK Consortium. 2012. Past Due: Remuneration and Social Protection for Caregivers in the Context of HIV and AIDS. Policy Brief, London, March. http://aidsconsortium.org.uk/wp-content/uploads/2011/11/UK-AIDS-Consoritum-policy-briefing-remuneration-of-caregivers.pdf.

UNAIDS. 2010. "State of the AIDS Response." Special Edition: Outlook. Geneva, UNAIDS.

Zimbabwe Evaluation Report. 2011a. *Social Capital and AIDS Competent Communities: Evidence from Eastern Zimbabwe.* Washington, DC: World Bank.*

———. 2011b. *Evaluation of Community Response to HIV and AIDS: Building Competent Communities: Evidence from Eastern Zimbabwe.* Washington, DC: World Bank.*

———. 2012. *Similarities and Differences in the Community Response to HIV and AIDS in Matabeleland South and Manicaland.* Washington, DC: World Bank.*

*See names of contributors to this report in appendix A.

Overview of Country Evaluation Cases

Abstract

Chapter 4 offers an overview of the country evaluation cases in Burkina Faso, India (2 evaluations of the impact of community responses on high risk groups, and one analytical study of programmatic shifts in the Avahan Program), Kenya (two evaluations of community responses), Lesotho (analysis of socioeconomic determinants of HIV stigma), Nigeria (evaluation of community responses), Senegal (evaluation of community responses and uptake of HIV counseling and testing), South Africa (evaluation of impact of peer and nutritional support on treatment adherence), and Zimbabwe (evaluation of the impact of grassroots organizations on HIV prevention, service utilization, and AIDS-related outcomes).

Introduction

This chapter summarizes the findings of each country evaluation. Table 4.1 depicts the areas studied in each of the countries. A short summary of the setting and findings is included after each evaluation. All information is taken from the Evaluation reports. See appendix D for further details of country evaluation cases.

Burkina Faso

Summary: This evaluation focused on the impact of community prevention activities on HIV/AIDS knowledge, behavior, and stigma. It found that although communities could be an effective vehicle for reducing stigma, there was a limited and mixed impact on knowledge, with effects varying by gender. The impact on behavior (including condom use and testing) appears to come from self-selection, resulting in a null result when an instrument for program exposure is used.

Country context: HIV/AIDS prevalence among adults in Burkina Faso was estimated at 1.6 percent (1.4–1.9) in 2007 by Joint United Nations Programme on HIV/AIDS (UNAIDS). Public action has been taken to limit the spread of the epidemic and mitigate its impact on health and welfare. Since 2001, Burkina

Table 4.1 Areas Reflected in Country Studies

	Burkina Faso	Kenya (HBCT)	India (FSW)	India (FSW MSM/T)	Kenya, Nigeria	Lesotho	Senegal	South Africa	Zimbabwe
Inputs for the community response									
Available resources for CBOs		✓			✓				✓
CBOs' workforce			✓		✓				✓
Characteristics of CBOs (qualitative analysis or components)				✓					
Effects of the community response on:									
Knowledge and behavior									
Knowledge of HIV	✓				✓				✓
Perceived HIV risk			✓	✓	✓				✓
Sexual risk behavior	✓		✓	✓	✓				✓
Activities and access to services									
Condoms use	✓		✓	✓	✓	✓			✓
STI		✓	✓	✓					
HIV testing	✓	✓			✓	✓	✓		✓
ART	✓	✓			✓	✓		✓	✓
Care					✓	✓			✓
PMTCT					✓	✓			✓

table continues next page

Table 4.1   Areas Reflected in Country Studies *(continued)*

	Burkina Faso	Kenya (HBCT)	India (FSW)	India (FSW MSM/T)	Kenya, Nigeria	Lesotho	Senegal	South Africa	Zimbabwe
Activities and social transformation									
Gender attitudes					✓	✓			
HIV/AIDS stigma	✓	✓	✓		✓	✓			✓
Attitudes towards PLWHA		✓			✓	✓			✓
Empowerment of communities			✓	✓					✓
OVC rights					✓	✓			
Social progress					✓				
Social capital					✓				✓
HIV incidence; other health outcomes									
HIV incidence				✓	✓				✓
STI prevalence				✓					✓

Sources: Burkina Faso Evaluation Report 2011; India Evaluation Report 2011, 2012a, 2012b; Kenya Evaluation Report 2011; Kenya HBCT Evaluation Report 2011; Nigeria Evaluation Report 2011; Senegal Evaluation Report 2010; South Africa Evaluation Report 2011; Zimbabwe Evaluation Report 2011a, 2011b, 2012.

Note: AIDS = acquired immune deficiency syndrome, ART = antiretroviral therapy, CBO = community-based organization, FSW = female sex worker, HBCT = home-based counseling and testing, HIV = human immunodeficiency virus, MSM/T = men who have sex with men and transgenders, OVC = orphans and vulnerable children, PLWHA = people living with HIV and AIDS, PMTCT = prevention of mother-to-child transmission, STI = sexually transmitted infection. Some themes were not studied in some countries.

Faso has implemented a national plan to fight HIV/AIDS, which has focused on decentralization and local community involvement. The creation of village committees to fight against HIV and AIDS (Comités Villageois de Lutte contre le VIH/SIDA) and the delivery of HIV and AIDS services by NGOs/CBOs illustrate this policy. The World Bank's Multi-Country HIV/AIDS Program (MAP) was also in place in Burkina Faso. Under the MAP, communities decided which prevention activity they would like to implement in accordance with the needs they identify. Communities then apply for funds and training from MAP before implementing the programs themselves.

Study focus: Interventions aimed at fighting HIV/AIDS can affect private and social behavior relating to the disease, such as sexual behavior; stigmatization of or tolerance toward HIV-positive individuals; communication about the disease among couples, families, and communities; and demand for voluntary counseling and testing services and antiretroviral treatment. The objective of the evaluation is to assess the effect of prevention activities on self-reported knowledge, sexual behavior, use of services, and stigma.

Methodology: The results are based on nationally representative data from 44,417 individuals in 8,496 households surveyed in Burkina Faso in 2007. Because individual participation may be endogenous, in addition to the survey results, the evaluation used individual's exposure to the community-based MAP program as an instrument for actual participation. In addition to avoiding the potential endogeneity bias, this contributes valuable information about community mobilization against HIV/AIDS as well as about self-selection issues.

Findings: Those who attended prevention activities reported significantly more desirable behavior than those who did not. Condom use, with one partner or the second one, was twice as high for those who attended prevention activities. On the other hand, fidelity and abstinence were less often reported by those who attended prevention sessions than by those who did not. This was likely due to people with more risky sexual behaviors being more apt to be interested in participating in HIV prevention activities. While participation in prevention is not significantly associated with less personal stigmatizing statements, it is associated with less stigmatization occurring in the community, as perceived and reported by respondent.

Using MAP exposure as an instrument, the analysis found that (a) exposure to prevention activities does not significantly increase knowledge about HIV/AIDS transmission mechanisms; (b) reported condom use with the first partner does not increase when exposed to a prevention program; and (c) program exposure may have a negative impact on HIV testing rates for men. However, the results on stigma are quite encouraging: living in a province where a MAP prevention program was implemented decreases the proportion of collective stigma by about 2 percentage points among both men and women as indicated by respondents. The community appears to play a role in making their members feel confident that the community would not reject infected people.

Conclusions: The general association of prevention and sexual behavior, knowledge about HIV/AIDS, and attitudes toward HIV-infected persons appears stronger when ignoring the issue of self-selection. The results suggest a strong self-selection of individuals attending prevention activities. Exposure to MAP did, however, have a significant effect on community-level stigma, suggesting that communities seem to make respondents feel more tolerant and amenable to taking action to help those infected by the virus. The null effect of MAP on condom usage and testing suggests that more focused interventions may be needed in this area.

India

Summary: Two evaluations in India looked at the impact of community response on high-risk groups, including female sex workers (FSWs) and men who have sex with men (MSM). The Andhra Pradesh study found that community collectivization was associated with increases in access to and utilization of health services and increased condom use by FSWs with partners. The Karnataka study found that empowerment of high-risk groups was associated with increased service utilization, condom usage, and effective social transformation.

Country context: India is experiencing a concentrated HIV epidemic. Moreover, there has been a steady decline in India's HIV prevalence rate from 0.45 percent in 2002 to 0.29 percent in 2008. An important factor accounting for this decline is the fall in the HIV prevalence rates among FSWs. According to a recent analysis, the decline in HIV prevalence among FSWs was estimated to result in a 36 percent reduction (2.7 million) of cumulative HIV cases by 2015.[1] Karnakata state and Andhra Pradesh state have the country's third and fourth highest prevalence rates: nearly 1 percent in Karnataka state and 1 percent among antenatal clinic attendees in Andhra Pradesh.[2] These characteristics—plus a government program that actively supports and regulates community engagement—motivated the focus of the evaluations in these states.[3]

Community mobilization has a long history in India. In the context of HIV and AIDS, it is viewed as one of the key mechanisms for containing the spread of the epidemic among groups at high risk of infections. Communities contribute by improving knowledge, reducing risky behavior, and stimulating access to health services. However, it is also recognized that significant obstacles are preventing groups at high risk of infection from exercising their own choices, applying safe sex practices, claiming their rights, and accessing health services. The objective of the two evaluation studies carried out in India was to develop a framework for measuring the empowerment process and evaluating its impact on various outputs and outcomes.

Karnataka State

The Karnataka State study was conducted in the context of a broad set of HIV prevention programs for FSWs in the state. It was implemented by the University of Manitoba and the Karnataka Health Promotion Trust (KHPT) as part of Avahan, the India AIDS Initiative of the Bill and Melinda Gates Foundation. The government is a major funder of civil society organizations (CSOs), especially those at the state and district level.

Study focus: The focus was on evaluating the results of the activities carried out under the Sankalp program that was launched in 2004. This program implemented comprehensive interventions to reduce risk and vulnerability among FSWs in 21 districts, covering more than 60,000 FSWs in a given year. To date, nearly 40,000 FSWs have enrolled in sex worker (SW) collectives, illustrating the substantial scale of community mobilization activities in the program.

Methodology: Several methods were used. One method aimed to report the ways in which various strategies of community mobilization impact domains of empowerment. Three indicators were developed to measure empowerment, and case studies were deconstructed into parts according to their impact on the various components of power and social context in the empowerment framework. Another method aimed to explore the relationship between community mobilization, empowerment, social transformation, and sexual health/HIV risk. Secondary analysis of three large surveys conducted in Karnataka from 2005 to 2010 by the researchers provided additional relevant information. These surveys included a behavioral tracking survey (BTS), and two rounds of integrated biological and behavioral surveys.

Findings: Regarding *access to and utilization of HIV-related services*, for all districts covered by the evaluation, *power within* was associated with the number of visits to health clinics during the previous 6 months.[4] Regarding *risk behavior*, greater empowerment, especially in the form of *power with*, was associated with increased condom use with occasional and regular clients.[5] On the *social transformation* front, all three domains of empowerment—power within, power with, and power over—were associated with intensity of program delivery at the district level.[6]

Membership in a community-based organization (CBO) was associated with reduced experience of violence, reduced police coercion, and an increased ownership of identity cards. It was also associated with reduced sexually transmitted infection (STI) in general, and reduced active syphilis in particular. HIV prevalence was also lower, but it was not statistically significant.

Conclusions: Based on this evidence, it would seem that FSW interventions may have had an impact on mitigating the epidemic in South India.

Andhra Pradesh State

The Andhra Pradesh State study examined community collectivization[7] and its association with outcomes among FSWs and high-risk men who have sex with men and transgenders (MSM/Ts). The program was implemented by the Hindustan Latex Family Planning Promotion Trust and the India AIDS alliance, Andhra Pradesh.

Study focus: The study dealt with two population groups in six districts, including 3,557 FSWs and 3,546 high-risk MSM/T. The key intervention was the community collectivization process, which includes community mobilization of high-risk groups; the building of an enabling environment; and engagement on issues of rights, entitlements, and stigma reduction.

Methodology: The evaluation used data from a BTS, a cross-sectional survey conducted during 2010/11 among FSWs and HR-MSM by the researchers. A framework was developed to measure the community collectivization process of FSWs and MSM/Ts and its impact on outcomes.

Findings for FSWs: Community collectivization of FSWs was found to increase access to and utilization of HIV-related services: the proportion of FSWs visiting a government health facility for STI treatment was significantly higher among those with medium versus low collectivization, 60.4 versus 42.4 percent. Community collectivization also significantly increased consistent condom use with occasional clients with increases in the degree of collectivization from low to high (74.5 versus 83.8 percent). Similar effects occurred with regular clients. Finally, it strengthened social transformation—FSWs who reported a high degree of collectivization compared to those who reported a low level of collectivization were more likely to believe in their own power to use condoms with clients and utilize services from government health facilities.

Findings for MSM/Ts: Community collectivization of MSM/Ts was found to (a) increase condom use with both paid partners (74.3 versus 48.1 percent) and nonpaying partners (73.5 versus 54.9 percent); (b) increase MSM/Ts' self-confidence to use condoms with clients and to express opinions (60.7 versus 50.9 percent); and (c) significantly increase consistent condom use with occasional clients with increases in the degree of collectivization from low to high (74.5 versus 83.8 percent). Similar effects occurred with regular clients. For MSM/Ts, community collectivization did not increase access to and utilization of government health facilities for STI treatment.

Conclusions: Among FSWs and MSM/T, community collectivization is predictive of condom use and ability to negotiate condom use.

Programmatic Shifts Analysis, Avahan Program

A new analysis of Avahan data based on a survey of nine community groups of FSWs and MSM in 2008–10 and 2009/10 showed that community group mobilization as measured by community ownership and preparedness, and participatory planning with NGOs and community groups resulted in (a) higher participation of the community in all aspects of program, (b) reductions in violence by police, (c) community response to crisis undertaken with no program involvement, (d) CBO awareness of laws relating to their rights and assumption of the primary role in negotiating for rights on behalf of communities of high-risk groups, and (e) CBOs working with other CSOs: women's, politicians', advocates', and media organizations.

Kenya

Summary: Two studies in Kenya examined the role of community response. The first was a comprehensive evaluation, including funding allocation, activities, and impacts. This study found that a stronger community response was associated with increased knowledge of HIV and lower-risk behavior. The second study was a randomized trial looking at the impact of home-based counseling and testing (HBCT) on stigma, which found that the intervention significantly decreased stigma among community leaders but did not have a strong impact on HIV knowledge.

Country context: Recent surveys estimate Kenya's HIV prevalence rate in the adult population to be between 7.4 percent (National AIDS Commission 2007) and 6.3 percent (National AIDS Commission 2008/09). The government recognized early on the importance of mobilizing civil society organizations, and especially CBOs, to strengthen the national AIDS response. Their involvement is a key component of the national response in the Kenya National AIDS Strategic Plan (KNASP III, 2009/10–2012/13) (National AIDS Commission 2009). However, the overall effects of their activities have not been rigorously assessed to date. To address this knowledge gap, the evaluation was conducted in Nyanza Province (HIV prevalence of 13.9 percent) and Western Province (HIV prevalence of 5.4 percent). These provinces have the highest prevalence rates in Kenya.

Community Response Study

Study focus: In recent years, several studies have evaluated the impact of specific activities conducted at the community level with the involvement of communities. Other studies have reported the main characteristics of community responses. However, there has been a general lack of robust evaluation of the community response viewed as a whole set of interventions. To assess the effects of the community response in Kenya, this evaluation aimed to determine whether a strong community response would generate better outcomes than a weaker community response with respect to (a) *HIV and AIDS-related results*—knowledge of prevention strategies, perceived HIV risk, and sexual risk behavior; (b) *utilization of HIV and AIDS-related services;* and (c) *social transformation results*—gender attitudes, HIV-related stigma, knowledge of orphans and vulnerable children (OVC) rights, and participation in political processes.

Methodology: The mixed-method evaluation used a quasi-experimental design, which consisted of three components: (a) a household survey carried out in 14 communities (7 study communities and 7 comparator communities); (b) qualitative data collected from CSOs and key informants; and (c) analysis of the allocation of funds data by CBOs. Communities demonstrating a stronger community response to HIV and AIDS were compared to communities with similar characteristics but showing a weaker response to HIV and AIDS. The strength of CBO engagement (a proxy for the community response) was measured by the percentage of households aware of CBO activities in their community. Communities demonstrating a *stronger* community response were assigned to the study group; those with a *weaker* community response were assigned to the comparison group.

Findings include the following:

- *Knowledge of HIV:* Study communities had better knowledge of HIV than comparison communities, including having one, uninfected partner (9 times better knowledge), using condoms (15 times better knowledge), and taking drugs to prevent mother-to-child transmission (4 times better knowledge). Virtually all CBOs indicated increasing AIDS-related knowledge and awareness among community members as their main achievements. Key informants also credited CBOs for these achievements.

- *Perceived risk:* Study communities had a higher perception of the risk of HIV infection.
- *Sexual risk behavior:* Study communities were four times more likely to use condoms consistently (with all sex partners during the past 12 months).
- *Use of HIV-related services:* There were no significant differences between the study and comparison communities as concerns HIV testing, use of treatment and care services and OVC-related support.
- *Gender attitudes and HIV-related stigma:* There was no indication that CBOs played a significant role concerning gender attitudes and HIV-related stigma. Other factors such as government policies, increased HIV awareness, and improvement in gender norms were mentioned by key informants.
- *Knowledge of OVC rights:* Study communities showed greater awareness of institutions that protect children's rights. However, key informants did not credit local CBOs with raising awareness.
- *Participation in political processes:* Study communities showed higher numbers of household members voting in national and local elections, as well as in participating in electoral campaigns.
- *CBO spending of resources:* Annual funding reported by the 25 CBOs surveyed averaged US$13,500 in the communities with high CBO engagement,[8] and US$7,506 in communities with low CBO engagement. In total, 46 percent of CBO funding came from bilateral and multilateral agencies. However, CBOs were able to mobilize support from a variety of sources, accessing funding from the central and local government as well as from private foundations and charities. CBOs in both communities also relied heavily on volunteer (paid and unpaid) support for service provision. As a result, CBOs may be increasing the total pool of funds available for the fight against AIDS in Kenya, rather than taking funding away from the central government.

Conclusions: The findings suggest that CBOs achieve results in addressing the HIV epidemic in specific ways that are closely tied to the services they provide. Thus, increasing CBO engagement can be an effective means for scaling up prevention efforts. At the same time, the evaluation findings suggest that these targeted prevention activities do not necessarily have a measurable impact on the larger social transformation indicators, such as HIV-related stigmatization and gender norms.

Home-Based Counseling and Testing Study

Study focus: The Academic Model Providing Access to Healthcare (AMPATH), a healthcare collaboration in western Kenya, provided home-based HIV counseling and testing to community members. Community leaders mobilized community members through road shows and town hall meetings to encourage HBCT uptake in advance of the testing event. Community leaders were educated about HIV/AIDS and the HBCT program and timeline. Facilitators, usually drawn from the local community, worked with local government to explain the HBCT program to the community. Locally based counselors visited all households in the community to provide voluntary counseling and offer testing to all adults. HIV tests and associated counseling were administered within the households, and couples were encouraged to test together. Finally, individuals who tested positive for HIV were referred to the local AMPATH treatment facility.

Methodology: A randomized control trial was adopted. Geographical locations were randomized to a study group receiving HBCT and a nonintervention control group receiving HBCT at a later date. Data were collected using a household survey in 2009 and 2011 ($n = 3,300$ individuals).

Findings include the following:

- HBCT and testing: HBCT was successful at increasing uptake of testing. The probability of testing rose by about 70 percent for those living in the treatment areas;
- HBCT and stigma: the evaluation found no negative relationship between stigma and levels of testing, which indicates that HBCT can be implemented with high rates of uptake, even in the presence of stigma;
- HBCT and risk behavior, HIV knowledge and reported condom use were not affected strongly or consistently;
- HBCT and social transformation, decreased stigmatization attitudes were evident among community leaders ($p < .05$). However, there were mixed effects on community members' stigmatization attitudes: HBCT decreased the sense that HIV was a sign of immoral behavior, but increased the feeling of anger and disgust towards those with HIV.

Conclusions: The study found that HIV knowledge and reported condom use were not affected by community mobilization, and the effects on stigmatization attitudes were unclear.

Lesotho

Summary: This study examined the relationship between HIV/AIDS stigma and take-up of services in a high prevalence area. HIV/AIDS stigma was strongly associated with a low probability of undergoing HIV tests and picking up test results, with men more easily deterred by stigma.

Country context: Lesotho has the third highest HIV prevalence rate in the world. The most recent estimates indicate an adult HIV prevalence of 23 percent, representing about 290,000 people living with HIV (PLHIV) (UNAIDS 2010). One of the key challenges in Lesotho is pervasive AIDS-related stigma. Stigmatizing beliefs about AIDS and associated fears of discrimination may be a barrier to the use of HIV-related services, such as HIV testing and counseling. The number of facilities providing HTC has increased and represents the largest share of expenditures on HIV prevention. However, most people in Lesotho still do not get tested. These issues motivated the design of the study.

Study focus: This study aimed to determine the socioeconomic determinants of HIV-related stigmatizing attitudes in Lesotho, and whether there is an association between fear of discrimination and the use of HIV testing services.

Methodology: Two consecutive rounds of the Lesotho Demographic and Health Survey were analyzed (Ministry of Health and Social Welfare Lesotho, Bureau of Statistics, and ORC Macro 2005; Ministry of Health and Social Welfare Lesotho and ICF Macro 2010). Data analysis focused on the percentages of women and men who express stigmatization attitudes toward PLHIV by background characteristics and the extent to which specific socioeconomic factors contribute to HIV stigmatization in women and men.

Findings: Stigmatizing attitudes related to AIDS were found to be associated with age (younger and older respondents were more likely to express discriminating behaviors than respondents 20–39 years old); gender (the proportion of respondents expressing stigmatizing attitudes was higher among men); lack of education; location (those living in urban areas were less likely to express discriminating behaviors); poverty (highest discriminating behavior was among the lowest wealth quintile); religion (different effects among men and women); and traditional circumcision.[9]

The study also found an association between fear of discrimination and use of HIV testing services as follows: (a) *Probability of being tested for HIV test (based on aggregate measure of stigmatization)*—HIV-related stigma is strongly associated with not using voluntary counseling and testing services. Men seem to be more easily deterred by the stigma of being tested for HIV; (b) *Probability of receiving HIV test results*—The higher the stigmatizing attitudes at the work place and within the household, the less likely that an individual obtains the result of an HIV test. For women, having some primary education has a positive effect on the likelihood of obtaining HIV test results.

Conclusions: The findings suggest that educational achievement (especially at the primary level), wealth, and an urban location are associated with less stigmatization. These findings underscore the importance of access to schooling and the need for effective HIV prevention programs in schools. Apart from the necessity to address HIV-related stigma from a human rights point of view, the Lesotho data also show that stigmatizing behaviors represent a barrier for HIV testing, and for obtaining the results of the test. As a result, policies to reduce stigma need to be incorporated into an effective HIV response.

Nigeria

Summary: This study was a comprehensive assessment of the community response to HIV. It was similar to the comprehensive Kenya study, focusing on funding allocation, activities, and impacts. In contrast to the Kenya study, though, this study found no effect on knowledge of HIV, perhaps because knowledge was already high. However, it did find a significant association of community response with access to and utilization of services. In this context, it found an impact of the use of services, especially in rural areas.

Country context: Although the overall adult HIV prevalence rate in Nigeria is 3.7 percent, it varies greatly by region (from 2.0 percent in the southwest to 7.0 percent in the south of the country). CSOs have emerged as a vital part of the HIV and AIDS response, especially the CBOs operating at the local level. The Civil Society Consultative Group on HIV/AIDS in Nigeria established in 2002 is a platform for NGOs and CBOs to participate in policy formulation.

Study focus: The focus of this evaluation was on assessing whether communities with a strong community response compared to communities with a weaker response show better outcomes in terms of (a) *HIV and AIDS-related results—* knowledge of HIV prevention strategies and sexual risk behavior; (b) *utilization of HIV and AIDS-related services;* and (c) *social transformation results—*gender attitudes, HIV-related stigma, knowledge of OVC rights, and social capital.

Methodology: Utilizing a quasi-experimental design, data were collected through a household survey in 28 communities. Qualitative data were collected from CBOs and key informants. Data were also collected through a funding allocation study with 35 CBOs in the study group and 19 CBOs in the comparison group. Twenty-eight communities were selected across six states that represent the geopolitical zones of Nigeria and that have the highest HIV-prevalence in their respective geopolitical zone. Communities were paired. Within each pair, the community with the higher number of CBOs relative to the population was considered to have a stronger community response and assigned to the study group; the community with the lower number of CBOs relative to the population was assigned to the comparison group. Households for survey were randomly selected.

Findings: (a) Seventy-seven percent of the CBOs studied engaged in some type of prevention efforts; (b) Thirty nine percent provided treatment and care, of which only a few provided HIV treatment including antiretroviral therapy (ART) (17 percent); (c) Forty two percent of care was in support for OVC; and (d) Seventeen percent was in impact mitigation. None of the interviewed CBOs conducted a systematic community needs assessment to inform their activities.

The strength of CBO engagement (number of CBOs per 100,000 inhabitants) was not associated with HIV/AIDS-related knowledge: respondents' demographic characteristics were better predictors of knowledge, as was condom use or the number of sex partners (in the previous 12 months). The strength of CBO engagement was not associated with reduced sexual risk behaviors. One reason may be that interviewed CBOs focused on education and information campaigns, and only a few reported engaging in targeted behavior change communication programs. As for AIDS-related morbidity and mortality rates, the strength of CBO engagement was not associated with the number of sick or deceased household members.

The impact of the community response on the access and use of AIDS and HIV-related services for CBOs was much greater in rural areas than in urban areas. An increase of 1 in the number of CBOs per 100,000 inhabitants was associated with (a) a more than twofold increase in the likelihood that a respondent would report using prevention services; (b) a 64 percent increase in the likelihood of reporting use of treatment; and (c) a 41 percent increase in the odds that an OVC received emotional or psychological support. In urban areas, the association between CBOs and service utilization was either weaker (such as for prevention), or, as was the case with treatment services and services provided to OVC, not statistically significant. Regarding gender attitudes, the strength of CBO engagement was not associated with the selected indicators of gender equality. The strength of CBO engagement was also not associated with the selected indicators of children's rights.

With respect to CBO funding, CBOs spent most on prevention services (25 percent of total expenditures) and socioeconomic impact mitigation, including support services for PLHIV and OVC (23 percent of total expenditures). Average annual funding levels were US$22,491 across organizations in the study group, and US$6,219 in the comparison group. Volunteers represented a substantial resource for CBOs, and CBOs devoted their funding to different activities than the national programs. Expenditures recorded in the National AIDS Spending Assessment (NASA) indicated that almost half of the funds in 2008 were spent on treatment and care (47 percent) and very little on impact mitigation and OVC support (2.5 percent). In contrast, the interviewed CBOs reported a much more equal allocation of funds among prevention, treatment and care, and impact mitigation.

Conclusions: The findings suggest that CBO engagement adds value to the national HIV response. The strength of CBO engagement was associated with increased service utilization, especially in rural areas. These findings are particularly encouraging as the availability of services by other types of organizations or the government is often limited in these locations. Consequently, further investment (that is, in funding and capacity building) in CBOs is needed, with an increased emphasis on those operating in rural areas. As there were already very high levels of knowledge and acceptance of PLHIV and low levels of reported stigma, no association was noted between the strength of CBO engagement and these indicators.

Senegal

Summary: This randomized study aimed to examine whether CBO activities could increase testing uptake in a concentrated epidemic area. The study found that peer mentoring was highly effective in increasing testing uptake, but traditional sensitization was not.

Country context: Senegal's epidemic is currently characterized as "stable" and "concentrated." The prevalence rate in the general population is low (0.9 percent) (UNAIDS 2010). Building on a tradition of social mobilization, the government quickly adopted a multisectoral approach, with several interventions taken to increase participation and representation. Civil society organizations have become increasingly involved in care and support activities. There are now more than 3,000 CSOs engaged in AIDS work in Senegal (Diouf 2007), ranging from local CBOs to larger national NGOs.

Study focus: HIV counseling and testing (HCT) sites are now widely available in Senegal in urban health facilities, as well as in rural health posts. However, HCT uptake remains extremely low (1.1 percent in 2007). This raises questions as to whether a peer-mentoring approach might be more effective than traditional social mobilization techniques. To answer this, an impact evaluation of peer mentoring took place in 2009/10, with the objective of comparing three types of programs delivered by CBOs: (a) traditional information campaigns on sexual behaviors and HIV; (b) standard social sensitization activities involving education about HIV and information about HCT, targeting a group of about 450 individuals drawn from the local communities; and (c) peer mentoring with peer education. The evaluation was aimed at assessing whether CBO programs are an effective way of increasing voluntary testing rates and/or changing the behavior of individuals who test positive, and whether the manner in which sensitization programs are delivered affects outcomes.

Methodology: This evaluation utilized a randomized approach, taking advantage of the phasing in of the peer-mentoring approach. Outcomes were measured by the data routinely collected at the administrative health district level. Participating CBOs were randomly allocated to one of three groups: (a) group 1 was the control group, CBOs that received no funding and provided traditional sensitization techniques (operating in 24 of 52 health districts); (b) group 2 was the first treatment group, CBOs that received funding and applied standard sensitization techniques (found in 9 health districts); and (c) group 3 was the second treatment group, CBOs that received funding and followed a peer-mentoring approach (in 19 health districts).

A total of 156,178 tests were given, with significantly more women tested than men. A relatively high proportion of individuals came back for their test results. In this data set, the average HIV prevalence rate was 4.7 percent. A Poisson regression model was used to test differences in outcome variables measured at the district level.

Study findings: Funding peer mentoring by CBOs increases the number of individuals who get tested compared to the control group (unfunded sensitization activities), whereas funded sensitization does not. Funded peer mentoring also increases the number of individuals who attend pre-test counseling, get tested, and who pick up their test results. These effects are mainly due to the increased number of women being tested. The number of individuals who access pre-test counseling, get tested, and pick up their test results increases by 100, 70, and 80 percent, respectively, due to peer mentoring.

Both peer mentoring and funded traditional sensitization activities significantly increase post-test counseling among individuals who test positive, with no statistically significant differences between peer mentoring and funded sensitization activities. These activities also increase the number of HIV-positive individuals whose partners have been tested.

Compared to unfunded sensitization activities, both peer mentoring and funded sensitization activities increase the number of HIV-positive individuals whose partners are tested. The effects of sensitization activities on HIV-positive individuals differ by gender: funded sensitization techniques are particularly effective in ensuring that infected women follow post-test counseling, whereas peer mentoring activities are particularly effective with men.

Conclusions: If the objective is to increase access to HCT services, funding peer mentoring activities is effective, whereas funding traditional sensitization techniques is not. Changing the behavior of HIV-positive individuals is more complex, and different approaches might be needed, especially as the effects vary by gender. Overall, although peer monitoring seems to be the most effective means of encouraging individuals to get tested for HIV and pick up their test results, funded sensitization campaigns seem to play a substantial role in modifying the behavior of infected individuals. This suggests that instead of focusing on one particular type of social mobilization technique, a combined approach is justified due to the complementarities of the different programs.

South Africa

Summary: This randomized study examined the impact of peer and nutritional support on treatment adherence in a generalized epidemic environment. It found that both forms of support reduced treatment delays.

Country/state context: South Africa faces the largest HIV burden in the world, with an estimated 5.3 million people living with HIV (UNAIDS 2010). Access to ART has expanded rapidly in South Africa, making it the country with the largest treatment program in the world. By February 2011, 1.4 million people were receiving ART, 95 percent in the public sector. As ART coverage continues to rise in resource-constrained settings, effective adherence support interventions are of central importance in ensuring the long-term sustainability of treatment.

Study focus: The objective of the evaluation was to assess the effects of peer and nutritional support on ART adherence. The evaluation looked at the Effective AIDS Treatment and Support in the Free State (FEATS) patient population, a prospective cohort study. In 2007/08, 648 adults who initiated ART in the past month were recruited into the FEATS study.

Methodology: Study participants were randomized to one of three treatment areas: (a) peer adherence support only, (b) peer adherence and nutritional support, and (c) a control group. Two rounds of follow-up interviews were conducted during the period March 2009 to July 2010. Multivariate fixed effects and instrumental variable regression models were employed to assess the impact of peer adherence and nutritional support interventions on self-reported adherence and timeliness of clinic and hospital visits.

Findings: After adjusting for potential endogeneity, selection bias, sociodemographic characteristics, and antiretroviral (ARV) treatment duration, delays in scheduled clinic visits for study participants visited twice weekly by a peer adherence supporter were statistically significantly lower than for study participants not receiving any peer adherence support. Delays in scheduled hospital visits were statistically significantly lower only for study participants receiving both adherence and nutritional support. Peer adherence and nutritional support had no significant impact on self-reported measures of adherence.

Conclusions: Preliminary results indicate that peer adherence and nutritional support improved the timeliness of adult clinic and hospital visits for routine follow-up while on ARV treatment. Further results are expected once the study is completed.

Zimbabwe

Summary: This evaluation used panel data to detect the impact of grassroots organization membership on HIV prevention, service utilization, and incidence over the 1999–2008 period. Community group participation with women was associated with increased prevention behaviors, higher service utilization, and, most important, lower HIV incidence. Benefits for men were not as significant. Overall, the effects of community response varied over time.

Country context: HIV prevalence in Zimbabwe peaked around 1997 at 26.5 percent, before falling steadily to 14.3 percent in 2009. Zimbabwe is one of the few countries in sub-Saharan Africa for which there is compelling evidence for substantial and sustained declines in HIV prevalence driven primarily by reductions in sexual risk behavior. The changes in behavior are believed to have been driven mainly by first-hand experience of AIDS illness and deaths among close friends and relatives, supported by scaled-up community-based HIV prevention programs. Interpersonal communication is thought to have played a key role in mediating the impacts of these factors on behavior. Despite these and other recent achievements, the HIV epidemic in Zimbabwe remains severe, especially in the Matabeleland province, which has the highest HIV prevalence rate, at 20.8 percent, followed by the Manicaland province, with 19.7 percent.

Study focus and methodology: Data covering the 1990–2008 period were used from a large-scale prospective general population cohort survey conducted in Manicaland province in eastern Zimbabwe. The data were analyzed to provide quantitative evidence regarding the contribution of community responses to the control of the HIV epidemic. Qualitative data, collected in parallel with the survey, were used to aid interpretation and to elaborate on the social processes that underlie the quantitative outcomes. A survey of CBOs provided information on funding and the allocation of resources in the Manicaland province.

Three specific questions were addressed in the study: (a) What forms of mobilization are associated with greater HIV avoidance and increased access to AIDS care and treatment? (b) What is the evidence for the causal pathways between community mobilization and health? (c) What are the community-level determinants of various types of intervention outcomes?

Findings: The community response to HIV/AIDS was found to have been extensive and to have had many positive effects. For women, participation in grassroots organizations (such as rotating credit groups, church groups, and burial societies) was associated with faster adoption of lower-risk sexual behavior and reduced HIV incidence during the late 1990s and early 2000s. Analysis of the 2003–08 data showed that women participating in community groups were quicker to take up new HIV services such as voluntary counseling and testing for HIV infection and prevention of mother-to-child transmission services. Benefits of group membership also extended to the entire community, which experienced lower HIV infection rates and a faster uptake of services.

Fewer positive effects were seen for men, in part because groups with different primary activities and characteristics differ in the effects they have on HIV-related outcomes. In addition, men tend to join groups whose activities and characteristics are less conducive to positive outcomes. As a consequence, in a few instances community participation was found to have negative outcomes.

The effects of community participation were found to have varied at different stages in the HIV epidemic. Findings suggest that community groups may play a useful role in accelerating the public response to a crisis or in offering the availability of a new service. However, once the threat has been fully recognized or a new program has become established, nongroup members may be equally likely to have responded or to have taken up the service.

Conclusions: Overall, women and men living in villages with greater community group membership were found to have improved outcomes, especially during the 1999–2003 period when the HIV and AIDS programs were substantially scaled up. These findings suggest that the protective effects of community groups are not permanent, but are perhaps best mobilized by introducing new programs. What is significant in a place such as Zimbabwe is precisely that CBOs/NGOs had this impact in the absence of a strong government response. This further highlights the critical role that CBOs/NGOs can play.

Overall Conclusions

In the portfolio of country cases, the impacts of community-based responses were found to be large and potentially crucial in ameliorating the worst effects of the AIDS epidemic in areas that may have been underserved by other forms of response. However, the success and impact of community responses were found to depend on a number of factors, such as how well suited the CBO or community groups focus was to the epidemic imperative and the needs expressed by the community, as well as the supporting environment of the response. The next chapter describes some of the key features of successful community responses.

Notes

1. Sex worker interventions were estimated to result in a 36 percent reduction (2.7 million) of cumulative HIV cases respectively by 2015 (National Evaluation of the AIDS Program 2008).

2. HIV sentinel surveillance and HIV estimation in India, 2007. National AIDS Control Organization, 2010.

3. See appendix D for more details on these studies.

4. *Power within* measured the degree to which the respondent did not feel ashamed to be identified as a FSW.

5. *Power with* measured the respondent's confidence in the ability of SWs to work together.

6. *Power over* measured social entitlement, for example, having a bank account.

7. Community collectivization was measured by three indicators: collective efficacy, collective agency, and collective action (see the three previous footnotes).

8. These data exclude one large CBO included in the sample.

9. Being circumcised is associated with higher stigmatization in men. In the Basotho culture, many young males are sent by parents to "initiation schools" where they are given information about sexual relations and reproductive health by elders. "Traditional circumcision" as a rite of passage into adulthood is more of a symbolic incision and differs from a medical circumcision.

References

Burkina Faso Evaluation Report. 2011. *Social and Individual Behaviour Change Initiated by Prevention Activities and Antiretroviral Treatment Provision in Burkina Faso.* Washington, DC: World Bank.*

Diouf, D. 2007. *HIV/AIDS Policy in Senegal: A Civil Society Perspective.* New York: Public Health Watch, Open Society Institute.

India Evaluation Report. 2011. *Evaluation of Community Mobilization and Empowerment in Relation to HIV Prevention among Female Sex Workers in Karnataka State, South India.* Washington, DC: World Bank.*

———. 2012a. *Using Data to Understand Programmatic Shifts in the Avahan HIV Prevention Program at the Community Level.* Washington, DC: World Bank.*

———. 2012b. *Community Collectivization and Its Association with Selected Outcomes among Female Sex Workers and High-Risk Men Who Have Sex with Men/Transgenders in Andhra Pradesh, India.* Washington, DC: World Bank.*

Kenya Evaluation Report. 2011. *Effects of the Community Response on HIV and AIDS in Kenya.* Washington, DC: World Bank.*

Kenya HBCT Evaluation Report. 2012. *The Links between Home-Based HIV Counseling and Testing and HIV Stigma in Western Kenya.* Washington, DC: World Bank.*

Lesotho Evaluation Report. 2011. *Combating the AIDS Pandemic in Lesotho by Understanding Beliefs and Behaviors.* Washington, DC: World Bank.*

Ministry of Health and Social Welfare (MOHSW) Lesotho, Bureau of Statistics (BOS) [Lesotho], and ORC Macro. 2005. *Lesotho Demographic and Health Survey 2004.* Calverton, MD: MOH, BOS, and ORC Macro.

Ministry of Health and Social Welfare (MOHSW) Lesotho, and ICF Macro. 2010. Lesotho *Demographic and Health Survey 2009.* Maseru, Lesotho: MOHSW and ICF Macro.

National AIDS Commission. 2007. *AIDS Indicators Survey.* Government of Kenya, Nairobi. http://www.nacc.or.ke/.

_____. 2008/09. *Demographic and Health Survey.* Government of Kenya, Nairobi. http://www.nacc.or.ke/.

_____. 2009. *Kenya National AIDS Strategic Plan (KNASP III, 2009/10–2012/13).* Government of Kenya, Nairobi. http://www.nacc.or.ke/.

Nigeria Evaluation Report 2011. *Effects of the Community Response to HIV and AIDS in Nigeria.* Washington, DC: World Bank.*

Senegal Evaluation Report. 2010. *HIV/AIDS Sensitization, Social Mobilization and Peer-Mentoring: Evidence from a Randomized Experiment.* Washington, DC: World Bank.*

South Africa Evaluation Report. 2011. *Timely Peer Adherence and Nutritional Support in Free State Province's Public Sector Antiretroviral Treatment Program.* Washington, DC: World Bank.*

UNAIDS (Joint United Nations Programme on HIV/AIDS). 2010. *State of the AIDS Response. Special edition, Outlook.* Geneva: UNAIDS.

Zimbabwe Evaluation Report. 2011a. *Social Capital and AIDS Competent Communities: Evidence from Eastern Zimbabwe.* Washington, DC: World Bank.*

———. 2011b. *Evaluation of Community Response to HIV and AIDS: Building Competent Communities: Evidence from Eastern Zimbabwe.* Washington, DC: World Bank.*

———. 2012. *Similarities and Differences in the Community Response to HIV and AIDS in Matabeleland South and Manicaland.* Washington, DC: World Bank.*

---

*See names of contributors to this report in appendix A.

CHAPTER 5

Features of Successful Community Responses

Abstract

Chapter 5 summarizes the main features of successful community responses. It describes the main characteristics of a "successful" community response as being affected by the types and stage of HIV epidemics; the alignment of community responses with AIDS responses; the legal, social and political environment provided by national policies; and the characteristics of communities and community organizations.

Introduction

Successful community responses depend on the type of HIV epidemic and the types and characteristics of community organizations, their links with government and other programs, and the wider legal, social, and political environment. The profile of a "successful" community response would be one where the local response (a) responds to the type and stage of the epidemic prevalent in the catchment area, (b) is aligned with the national response goals and priorities, (c) supports and contributes to other national programs to address the multisectoral nature of AIDS, and (d) is supported and protected by national policies. The first point is particularly relevant. Embedded in the concept of being "responsive to the epidemic" are the attributes of better targeting of services and actions, reaching those most at risk and affected by the epidemic, as well as better focused interventions with realistic expectations. Finally, the characteristics of the communities themselves play a role.

Type and Stages of HIV Epidemics

The community response was generally viewed as most appropriate in the context of high HIV prevalence and generalized epidemics, as the engagement of the whole society was needed to reverse the course of the HIV epidemic (UNAIDS 2007). This was the case in Zimbabwe, where the community response was found to be strong enough to reduce HIV infections.

In other types of HIV epidemics, there were questions concerning the role of community responses. This evaluation shows that they can have a substantial role. In a concentrated epidemic such as that in India, community mobilization of female sex workers (FSWs) was shown to be effective in improving biological outcomes. In other contexts, the examples of Burkina Faso, Kenya, and Nigeria suggest that the community response can affect some components of the chain of results from inputs to outcomes, but it does not seem strong enough to affect all of the components. Nevertheless, the community response contributes to attaining specific goals of the national response.

The effects of the community response may also depend on the stage of the HIV epidemic. The role of communities is likely to be stronger during the stage when a large share of the population is affected by AIDS-related deaths and comorbidity, and when people have strong incentives to protect themselves from infections. Zimbabwe provided such an example in the late 1990s. In later stages of the epidemic, as knowledge about the epidemic becomes more widespread and behavioral changes extend throughout the population, there are presumably much smaller differences between those who were members of a community group and those who were not. As a result, in this later stage of the HIV epidemic, group membership may provide a much weaker protective role. Thus, as the epidemic evolves, community groups might need to reorient themselves in order to maintain their protective role. One example could be to promote other behaviors, such as treatment adherence or voluntary male circumcision.

Alignment and Linkages with the AIDS Response

Strong links between the community and national responses can help increase the effectiveness of the community response. This can take the form of a framework that guides the activities of community-based organizations (CBOs) and small nongovernmental organizations (NGOs), as evidenced by the India, Kenya, and Nigeria examples. In India, the activities of small NGOs and CBOs are guided by a set of standardized interventions that have been defined by the National AIDS Control Program (NAC III). Over 1,600 targeted interventions covering 1.1 million high-risk groups are being implemented by 2,200 small NGOs and CBOs. In Kenya and Nigeria, the community response figures prominently in their governments' national AIDS strategic plans. CBOs receive funding in support of specific targeted activities. In such a context, the community response can effectively complement the national response.

Links with other national programs: Success can also be increased through strong links with governmental health facilities and social services. Faced with small budgets, CBOs cannot provide services in all areas of the continuum of services from prevention to treatment, care, and support. However, they can increase community access to and use of services by creating demand and providing referrals. To ensure that CBOs can play this role, government ministries might have to provide adequate training to CBO staff and/or volunteers and make clear how CBOs can best help—that is, what specific results they would help to achieve.

Government and donor programs can also trigger community responses. The Avahan program in India provided incentives, while the motivation of community members helped create strong empowerment among FSWs and men who have sex with men and transgenders[1] (MSM/Ts) and encouraged communities to take an increasingly autonomous role (India Evaluation Report 2012a). When new programs are being introduced to expand the HIV response, they create a burst of enthusiasm that can help energize community responses. This was the case in Zimbabwe in the early 2000s when the HIV response was being expanded to deal with the epidemic.

National Policies in Support of Community Action: Legal, Social, and Political Environment

A strong tradition of grassroots organizations, a favorable legal environment, and a participatory local government can facilitate the involvement of CBOs in the HIV response. In Zimbabwe, a variety of community groups were already part of community life when the epidemic emerged. They provided a readily available space for discussing HIV- and AIDS-related issues. In India, the legal and social environment for commercial sex work was repressive, but it allowed FSWs to form groups. However, this did not occur to the same extent for MSM/Ts as they faced a much more repressive environment. In Kenya, changes in laws were mentioned by key informants as the most important factor explaining increased awareness of women's rights and decreased violence against women.

Characteristics of Communities and Community Organizations

Relevant characteristics of communities that matter include the community structures and types of organizations, the ownership of programs, the amount of resources and their use, their target groups, and their role in supporting broader government programs. In Zimbabwe, the protective effects of membership for the general population varied across groups. The most effective ones were observed when grassroots groups provided members with a space for interpersonal exchange of information and discussion of HIV-related issues. In India, groups formed by FSWs and MSM/Ts provided the same function, as well as a means for implementing social changes (e.g., a reduction in police violence).

Types of Organizations

A substantial percentage of community structures and CBOs are faith based. One advantage of these groups is that they have access to philanthropic funds. Some of these funds directly support national priorities; others are focused more on meeting local needs of a broad nature. According to this evaluation, CBOs received about 25 percent of their funding through philanthropy.

In analyzing a civil society organization (CSO) dataset collected by Birdsall and Kelly (2007), Olivier and Wodon (2012) find that out of 349 organizations running HIV and AIDS programs in Southern Africa, 117 were faith based and 232 were secular. For both groups, 55 percent of the CSOs are located in a town or city that serves as an administrative center for surrounding areas or towns, and 45 percent are in a rural village or small town. For both groups, close to three-fourths of CSOs work in more than one community. The number of years of existence of the CSOs and of experience in working on HIV and AIDS is also similar for both types of CSOs.

There are, however, a few areas where one observes differences between the two types of CSOs. The proportion of faith-inspired CSOs that have branches or programs in other countries, at 18 percent, is higher than for secular CSOs, at 10 percent. The proportion of faith-inspired CSOs that are part of an HIV/AIDS association or coordinating network/body is also slightly higher, at 90 percent, than for secular CSOs, at 83 percent. Also, 72 percent of faith-inspired CSOs conduct activities not related to HIV/AIDS, versus 64 percent of secular CSOs. This suggests that at least in the sample of relatively large CSOs, as opposed to the smaller ones working in only one community, faith-inspired CSOs tend to be slightly more international, connected to other organizations working on HIV/AIDS, and active in other areas than is the case for secular CSOs. Another difference between the two types of organizations is that, as expected, secular CSOs tend to have a higher ratio of paid staff (full-time or part-time) to the number of volunteers working for the organization than is the case for faith-inspired CSOs. This is true for both national and international staff.

Community Ownership of Programs

A case study of two randomized control trials in Zimbabwe (Zimbabwe Evaluation Report 2011) brings out the role that community ownership and involvement (or lack thereof) can have on program outcomes. The first one is a 1998–2003 community randomized controlled trial carried out to evaluate the feasibility and impact of peer education, condom distribution, income-generating projects, and clinic-based STI treatment and counseling services in eastern Zimbabwe among persons engaging in commercial sex. Results showed no statistically significant impact on HIV incidence. The second study (2009–11) is another community randomized controlled trial to evaluate the impact of providing bimonthly cash transfers to households caring for orphans and vulnerable children (OVC) on the well-being of these children. Preliminary findings are encouraging. Under the first study, there was a poor fit between the externally funded program goals, messages, methods, and local communities' perceptions and realities. These lessons were applied in the second program design and explain the much better endorsement of the program by communities. Similarly, the success of the empowerment program of FSWs and MSM/Ts in India seems to be related to a systematic policy of empowering these groups so that they can pursue their own community agendas beyond the lifetime of the Avahan program (India Evaluation Reports 2011, 2012a, 2012b).

Mobilization and Use of Resources

Successful community responses depend on resources in the form of funding and human resources, mainly volunteers. On average, CBOs located in communities with strong engagement by community groups, such as in Kenya and Nigeria, mobilized more resources and showed better results than CBOs in communities with weaker community engagement. More active communities attract more resources. However, the use of these resources matters. Successful community responses are those in which funding is allocated to areas where it can have an impact. In several cases, however, there is no indication that community organizations did a systematic assessment of needs. Instead, the availability of external funding was the critical if not the only factor that guided the activities of CBOs.

Group Targeting by Gender
The effects of community responses are not gender neutral. Some types of communication outreach are more effective among women, whereas others are more effective among men. For instance, group membership was found to benefit women in Zimbabwe but did not benefit men. However, certain types of support groups, especially peer support for ART treatment in South Africa and peer sensitization for HTC in Senegal, are beneficial to men.

Support of National Programs
As discussed, communities benefit when they have positive links with national programs and are included in the national response to HIV and AIDS. Such links often result in the ability of communities to access funds and obtain support for technical capacity building. Sometimes this is facilitated by national CBO networks that ensure direct donor or government funding and then support communities in implementing specific programs and actions.

The findings of this evaluation identify many of the results achieved by communities and CBOs, pointing to a natural complementarity between community response and government actions. It would seem then that civil society remains as relevant now as it was in the early days of the urgent AIDS crisis. As the findings show, community groups and CBOs are still playing a crucial role, and their importance has not diminished as the government and external response has expanded. The role of the community response would need to adapt as the epidemic evolves and the priority actions shift toward treatment and biomedical interventions such as male circumcision, but communities can still be a very important service delivery mechanism and prevention agent.

All of these characteristics of successful community responses point to the potential for less risky behaviors, a culture of support, better use of prevention and treatment and care facilities, and the increased likelihood that both individuals and community groups will offer support to those affected by AIDS. These are important benefits that strengthen the overall impact of national AIDS responses. This is why evaluating community responses is important. As strategies for the mainstreaming of HIV services are being considered, these features would be relevant to programming and implementation. The overall findings of this evaluation point to areas where community groups can better achieve results.

The overarching message relates to the need to continue building a strong pool of evidence and to use such evidence in support of sound decision making to ameliorate the HIV and AIDS epidemic.

Note

1. The Avahan program was funded by the Bill and Melinda Gates Foundation.

References

Birdsall, K., and K. Kelly. 2007. *Community Responses to HIV/AIDS in South Africa: Findings from a Multi-Community Study.* Johannesburg: Centre for AIDS Development, Research and Evaluation (CADRE).

India Evaluation Report. 2011. *Evaluation of Community Mobilization and Empowerment in Relation to HIV Prevention among Female Sex Workers in Karnataka State, South India.* Washington, DC: World Bank.*

India Evaluation Report. 2012a. *Using Data to Understand Programmatic Shifts in the Avahan HIV Prevention Program at the Community Level.* Washington, DC: World Bank.*

India Evaluation Report. 2012b. *Community Collectivization and Its Association with Selected Outcomes among Female Sex Workes and High-Risk Men Who Have Sex with Men/Transgenders in Andhra Pradesh, India.* Washington, DC: World Bank.*

Olivier, J., and Wodon Q. 2012. *Who Benefited from Increased Funding on HIV/AIDS in Africa? Comparing Faith-Based and Non-religious Organizations.* Washington, DC: World Bank.

UNAIDS (Joint United Nations Programme on HIV/AIDS). 2007. *Practical Guidelines for Intensifying HIV Prevention: Towards Universal Access.* Geneva: UNAIDS.

Zimbabwe Evaluation Report. 2011. *Social Capital and AIDS Competent Communities: Evidence from Eastern Zimbabwe.* Washington, DC: World Bank.*

*See names of contributors to this report in appendix A.

Conclusion and Recommendations

Abstract

Chapter 6 summarizes the key contributions that communities can make to national AIDS responses as well as the limitations of community responses. It indicates the main implications for designing effective community responses as concerns civil society organizations, governments and donor agencies.

Introduction

The evaluation studies synthesized in this document were carried out to provide a better understanding of the community response, its contribution to halting the HIV epidemic, and its role in mitigating the epidemic's impact. The studies, which collected primary data, sought to answer whether a strong community response resulted in better HIV-related outcomes—that is, utilization of relevant services; knowledge, attitudes, behaviors; HIV-related impact measures; and social transformation. Taken individually, each study provides a partial view and sometimes limited evidence that the community response influences knowledge, behavior, and the use of services. Taken in their totality, however, the studies provide a robust knowledge base that community mobilization can deliver positive results.

Evaluation Summary

This evaluation details the various contributions that communities have made, including the following:

- A strong community response provides benefits that range from increased knowledge, to changed behavior, to increased use of services in the context of high HIV prevalence epidemics.
- The increase in access to services is especially evidenced among the most at-risk and marginalized populations and when it is targeted to specific groups and focused on specific services.
- In the context of geographically mixed epidemics, the community response helps increase the demand for government services by informing the

community about services, supporting the community's use of those services, and providing referrals.

- The community response is critical in servicing hard-to-reach populations, such as those in rural areas. This points to some of the crucial roles that community-based organizations (CBOs) can and do play. In this context, the community response has an advantage over other service providers, such as extension workers, who work *in* communities but may not be *of* the community.
- CBOs can do much with little. A small budget goes a long way. Supporting community groups and CBOs to work not only hard, but also smart, has the potential for improving community-based activities and for accruing tangible results on investments.

The community response contributes to national responses to HIV and AIDS through different pathways. For example, they can help increase HIV knowledge and inform community members about HIV services and AIDS treatment as well as promote the use of health services, thereby achieving better health outcomes. India provides an example of such a positive pathway in the case of female sex workers (FSWs). The evidence from the evaluation of peer support on HIV testing is strong (causal evidence in Senegal). However, the role of peer support on adherence showed mixed effects. Peer support improved the timeliness of clinical visits in South Africa, but the effect on actual adherence was weak. This result adds to the mixed picture of community-based adherence support provided by recent systematic reviews, with one systematic review finding no effect (Ford et al. 2009) and another reporting positive effects (Hart et al. 2010). Understating the factors that affect antiretroviral therapy (ART) adherence would be critical for defining a clear role for communities in this area and to improving and sustaining results.

Another pathway involves a direct effect of community mobilization in reducing risk behaviors and ultimately HIV infections, as happened in Zimbabwe during the late 1990s. This pathway may be less costly than the other pathway involving access to services. In countries, where the labor cost of community members may be low, the strengthening of community groups could be a cost-effective way of reducing infections. However, this proposition would need to be supported by further analysis specifically focusing on the cost-effectiveness aspects of community responses.

The evaluation also reveals the limitations of the community response—the means by which to measure it.

First and foremost, the impact of the community response cannot be guaranteed, as it is likely to vary among countries. For instance:

- At the time of this evaluation, strong CBO engagement resulted in very different effects on knowledge and the use of services in Kenya and Nigeria, mainly because of the differences in existing HIV knowledge levels in each country as well as differences in CBO activities' alignment with the national AIDS response and epidemic priorities.

- In Zimbabwe, the effects of the community response were much stronger during the initial phase of the epidemic (1998–2003), when new programs were being introduced, than in later years.
- Limited evidence was found that community response affects broader social changes in the context of low-HIV prevalence countries (Kenya and Nigeria). However, community impacts on social changes were demonstrated in the India studies, particularly for FSWs and men who have sex with men and transgenders (MSM/T).
- Unexpected adverse results were found in a number of cases, especially concerning stigmatization—an area with unclear results across the board.

Still, there is enough corroborating evidence to enable the application of these findings to improve the results of the HIV and AIDS response. The implications of the findings have been presented in detail in the executive summary. This chapter discusses broader considerations for dialogue and debate, which are linked to the implications already presented.

On the broad policy and programmatic fronts, decision makers need to consider the strengths and also the limitations intrinsic to community responses. Communities or CBOs cannot do everything. A community response cannot become a substitute for weak national responses, but communities can help deliver specific results.

Thus, programs will benefit from restraint—that is, shifting efforts to the achievement of clear, specific, manageable, and realistic expectations at the community level, even if this means having fewer goals.

- In concentrated epidemics, population groups at higher risk of infection can be empowered and mobilized to change behavior, a process that has the potential of reducing infections. This is a qualitative process, and thus policy makers may wish to consider well-focused qualitative approaches to support achieving specific desired outcomes.
- In a context where the epidemic is generalized, a broader, more comprehensive portfolio of community-based activities may be needed to achieve the wider social and cultural changes that are required for reversing the course of the epidemic.
- Community groups such as caregivers and CBOs can deliver valuable services, provided they are focused on specific activities that can complement national and intranational HIV and AIDS priorities (e.g., advocacy combined with referrals to services), filling gaps in local responses (e.g., in underserved areas), or offering innovative approaches.
- In all cases, ownership of community responses by their members needs to be sustained, especially in the case of donor-funded projects. There is no straight path toward that goal. However, funders may want to follow participatory

approaches to assess needs, involve community members in the design of projects to ensure ownership and stronger consistency with social customs, and build the capacity of communities to take over the management of projects.

The community response needs better-focused support that takes into account the different roles of community groups depending on the context.

- Funding that is directed to priority areas and proven HIV and AIDS programs, such as for FSWs, or to innovative approaches for men who have sex with men (MSM) is more likely to yield results. There is robust evidence that sex-work-driven epidemics are preventable—perhaps the single most successful prevention intervention. They are also effective interventions for MSM, but new and creative approaches are needed to overcome obstacles in repressive environments. Thus, community-based activities can potentially complement rather than duplicate government or others services.

- Within the existing funding envelopes at the national and global levels, there needs to be an effort to channel more funding to the community level. One way to optimize such funding would entail exploring different funding mechanisms that are more closely linked to achieving concrete results, such as performance-based contracting or cash transfers. Approaches such as these have embedded in them clear performance expectations and indicators. For instance, linking public health sector services with CBOs would create purposeful partnerships with community-based providers to facilitate patient care and referrals.

- Issues of efficiency and effectiveness are critical but need to be considered within the contextual reality of where CBOs and other community groups work. Many do so in remote areas, working with disadvantaged populations. In this context, issues of equity would be important to consider. Improving allocative efficiency would be a critical first step. This could be achieved by prioritizing areas for funding and program implementation, and reducing gaps and overlaps in funding coverage. For example, in several of the countries studied, CBO activities are not taking place in areas that are essential for reversing the course of the epidemic and/or they are duplicating other national HIV and AIDS programs.

- Donors face an inherent trade-off between obtaining quick and monitorable results versus a longer-term process of institution building that may or may not lead to more effective community responses. The first objective is most easily achieved by funding large international or national nongovernmental organization (NGOs) that then supervise community groups to implement projects. However, these projects may not be sustainable once external assistance ceases. Institution building can strengthen the sustainability of the community response, but it requires a longer time commitment. Some areas for consideration would include (a) establishing funding channels to facilitate access of community groups and CBOs to funding, while at the same time strengthening their capacity to collect and report data on costs, budgets, and activities; (b) providing technical support that is targeted to enabling the implementation of specific community-based activities, including standards of practice, normative materials, related training, and links to civil society networks and government agencies; and (c) supporting the role of caregivers and "volunteers" with compensation, remuneration, training, or other incentives.

National and international civil society networks and alliances are critical to support community responses. Civil society organizations (CSOs) have traditionally been viewed as providers of humanitarian assistance, as representatives of the voices of vulnerable or marginalized groups, and as social advocates and innovators. These different roles were encountered in the country evaluations of the community response. As the epidemic evolves and the HIV mainstreaming dialogue becomes more prevalent, civil society has an opportunity to be part of the dialogue and influence its outcomes. This might mean that roles and responsibilities may need to shift to ensure that the needs of communities in a changing fiscal and social environment are served.

The community response cannot be taken for granted, nor can it be guaranteed. A certain community-fatigue could be looming on the horizon—triggered by ever-increasing needs, decreasing resources, and changing priorities. Yet the global HIV goals cannot be achieved without the participation of communities.

References

Ford, N., J. B. Nachega, M. E. Engel, and E. J. Mills. 2009. "Directly Observed Antiretroviral Therapy: A Systematic Review and Meta-Analysis of Randomized Clinical Trials." *Lancet* 374: 2064–71.

Hart, J. E., C. Y. Yean, L. C. Ivers, H. L. Behforouz, A. Caldas, P. C. Drobaca, and S. S. Shin. 2010. "Effect of Directly Observed Therapy for Highly Active Antiretroviral Therapy on Virologic, Immunologic and Adherence Outcomes: A Meta-Analysis and Systematic Review." *Journal of Acquired Immune Deficiency Syndromes* 54 (2): 167–79.

Evaluation Teams and List of Study Reports

Abstract

Appendix A lists the evaluation teams and study reports, broken down by region.

Introduction

The research teams responsible for the evaluation studies as well as the authors of evaluations reports are listed below. This evaluation could not have been done without the experience, skills, and commitment of researchers and national authorities in the different countries. To all, we express our sincere appreciation.

World Bank Evaluation Team

Rosalía Rodriguez-García, René Bonnel, N'Della N'Jie, and Brian Pascual, with Damien de Walque, Markus Goldstein, Ariana Logovini, and Uma Balasubramanian and Mario Mendez.

Country Evaluation Teams and Reports

Burkina Faso

The Burkina Faso evaluation, *Social and Individual Behavior Change Initiated by HIV/AIDS Prevention Activities*, was prepared by Damien de Walque, Harounan Kazianga, Mead Over, and Elisa Rothenbuhler. 2011.

India

The India evaluation report for Karnataka State, *Evaluation of Community Mobilization and Empowerment in Relation to HIV Prevention among Female Sex Workers in Karnataka State, South India*, was prepared by H. L. Mohan, A. K. Blanchard, M. Shahmanesh, R. Prakash, S. Isac, B. M. Ramesh, P. Bhattacharjee, and S. Moses. 2011.

The India evaluation report for Andhra Pradesh, *Community Collectivization and Its Association with Selected Outcomes among Female Sex Workers and High-Risk Men Who Have Sex with Men/Transgenders in Andhra Pradesh, India*, was prepared by Niranjan Saggurti, Ram Manohar Mishra, Laxminaryana Proddutoor, Saroj Tucker, Dolly Kovvali, Prabhakar Parimi, and Tisha Wheeler. 2012.

The India background paper *Using Data to Understand Programmatic Shifts in the Avahan HIV Prevention Program at the Community Level* was prepared by Pradeep Narayanan, K. Moulasha, Tisha Wheeler, James Baer, and Tom Thomas. 2012.

Kenya

The Kenya evaluation report *Effects of the Community Response on HIV and AIDS in Kenya* was prepared by a team (a) from the National AIDS Control Council—Professor Alloys Orago, Sobbie Mulindi, Patrick Muriithi, and Ben Mundia; (b) from ICF Macro—Kara Riehman, Brigitte Manteuffel, Jakub Kakietek, and Joseph Fruh; (c) from the Kenyan National Coordinating Agency for Population and Development (NCAPD)—Paul Kizito and Vane Lumumba; and (d) from the World Bank—Rosalía Rodriguez-García, René Bonnel, N'Della N'Jie, Katie Bigmore, and Wacuka Ikua. 2011.

The Kenya study report *The Links between Home-Based HIV Counseling and Testing and HIV Stigma in Western Kenya* was prepared by Markus Goldstein, Corinne Low, Samson Ndege, Cristian Pop-Eleches, and Harsha Thirumurthy. 2012.

The Kenya analytical study *Evaluating the Structure of the Costs of Community-Based Organizations Involved in the Community Response to HIV and AIDS in Kenya* was prepared by Bruce Larson of Boston University. 2012.

Lesotho

The Lesotho evaluation report *Combating the AIDS Pandemic by Understanding Beliefs, Behaviors, and Stigmatizing Attitudes,* was prepared by Lucia Corno and Damien de Walque. 2011.

The Lesotho evaluation report *Community Responses to HIV/AIDS: A Retrospective Qualitative Review* was prepared by Damien de Walque and Rachel Kline. 2011.

Nigeria

The Nigeria evaluation report *Effects of the Community Response to HIV and AIDS in Nigeria* was prepared by a team: (a) from the National Agency for the Control of AIDS: Professor John Idoko, Kayode Ogungbemi, James Anenih, Akinrogunde, and Ronke Adeoye; (b) from the National Population Commission: Sani ali Gar, Inuwa Jalingo, Osifo T. Ojogun, David Fasiku, Bintu Ibrahim, and S.M.O Unogu; (c) from ICF Macro: Jakub Kakietek, Tesfayi Gebreselassie, Brigitte Manteuffel, Anna

Krivelyova, Sarah Bausche, and Joseph Fruh, and (d) from The World Bank: Rosalía Rodriguez-Garcia, René Bonnel, N'Della N'Jie, Michael O'Dwyer, and Francisca Ayodeji Akala. 2011.

The Nigeria evaluation report *Secondary Analysis of Data from the Evaluation of the Community Response to HIV and AIDS in Nigeria by State* was prepared by ICF Macro. 2012.

Senegal

The Senegal evaluation report, *HIV/AIDS Sensitization, Social Mobilization and Peer Mentoring: Evidence from a Randomized Experiment* (working title), was prepared by Jean-Louis Arcand, Pape Alioune Diallo, Cheikhou Sakho, Natasha Wagner, P. Slioune, and Arianna Legovini. 2010 draft.

South Africa

The South Africa evaluation report, *Peer Adherence and Nutritional Support in Free State Province's Public Sector Antiretroviral Treatment Programme*, was prepared by Frikkie Booysen, Damien de Walque, Mead Over, Sakoto Hashimoto, and Chantell de Reuck. 2011.

Zimbabwe

The Zimbabwe evaluation report *Evaluation of Community Responses to HIV and AIDS, Building Competent Communities: Evidence from Eastern Zimbabwe* was prepared by Simon Gregson, Constance Nyamukapa, Lorraine Sherr, and Catherine Campbell. 2011.

The Zimbabwe qualitative research report *Social Capital and AIDS Competent Communities: Evidence from Eastern Zimbabwe* (draft) was prepared by Catherine Campbell, Kerry Scott, Mercy Nhamo, Kate Morley, Constance Nyamukapa, Claudius Madanhire, Morten Skovdal, Lorraine Sherr, and Simon Gregson. 2011 draft.

The Zimbabwe evaluation report *Similarities and Differences in the Community Response to HIV and AIDS in Matabeleland South and Manicaland* (draft) was prepared by Morten Skovdal, Sitholubuhle Magutshwa-Zitha, Catherine Campbell, Constance Nyamukapa, and Simon Gregson. 2011.

The Zimbabwe Evaluation Team includes the following: (a) from Imperial College, London, Simon Gregson and Constance Nyamukapa; (b) from the London School of Economics, Catherine Campbell, Kerry Scott, Mercy Nhamo, Morten Skovdal, and Kate Morley; (c) from the Biomedical Research and Training Institute, Harare, Constance Nyamukapa, Claudius Madanhire, Isaiah Abureni, Simon Gregson, Busani Gwesela, Sitholubuhle Magutshwa-Zitha, Norman Mapani, Ncedani Ncube, Nkululeko Ncube, Mercy Nhamo, Monalisa Nhengu, and Stewart Rupende; (d) from the University of Bergen, Morten Skovdal; (e) from University College, London, Lorraine Sherr; (f) from the National AIDS Commission, Freeman Dube, Tapuwa Magure, and Raymond Yekeye; (g) from the World Bank, Rosalía Rodriguez-García, René Bonnel, and N'Della N'Jie.

Desk Studies and Background Papers

Efficacy of Community-Based Organizational Input on Supporting Orphans and Vulnerable Children (OVC) Outcomes in Relation to HIV 2004–2009: OVC; A Systematic Review, prepared by Lorraine Sherr. 2010 background paper.

A Survey of Stakeholders to Identify the "Lenses" to Approach the Community Response Evaluation, prepared by Roger Drew. 2010 background paper.

"Analyzing Community Responses to HIV and AIDS: Operational Framework and Typology," prepared by Rosalía Rodriguez-García, René Bonnel, N'Della N'Jie, Jill Olivier, F. Brian Pascual, and Quentin Wodon. *World Bank Policy Research Working Papers* # 5532. 2011.

Funding Mechanisms for the Community Response to HIV and AIDS, prepared by René Bonnel, Rosalía Rodriguez-Garcia, Jill Olivier, Quentin Wodon, Sam McPherson, Kevin Orr, and Julia Ross. 2011 background paper.

Flow of Resources in Community-Based Organizations in Kenya, Nigeria, and Zimbabwe, was prepared by Jakub Kakietek. 2012 field/desk study.

Country Briefs and Evaluation Summaries

Country briefs on Burkina Faso, Kenya, Lesotho, Nigeria, Senegal, and Zimbabwe; summary of evaluation findings; and other materials can be found on the UK Consortium on AIDS and International Development website: *aidsconsortium .org.uk.*

Peer Consultations

Abstract

Appendix B lists the peer reviewers, broken down by continent.

Peer Reviewers

We wish to express our appreciation to those peer reviewers who provided valuable comments and suggestions to previous versions of the final report, and many more who took the time during the process of this evaluation to review and contribute their experiences and insights. By so doing, they made all the products of this evaluation better. (Our sincere apologies if we have missed anyone.) These include institutions in alphabetical order:

Africa

Centre for Health Policy and Innovation (IDRC), South Africa—Marco Gomes
Eastern African National Network of AIDS Service Organizations (EANNASO), Tanzania—Titus James Twesige
Kenya AIDS NGO Consortium—Rosemary Mburu
Southern Africa HIV and AIDS Information Dissemination Service (SAfAIDS)—Sara Page-Mtongwiza and Lois Chingandu
The AIDS Consortium, South Africa—Denise Hunt
United Nations Children's Fund Eastern and Southern Africa Regional Office—Thomas H. Fenn
World YWCA—Nyaradzayi Gumbonzvanda

Asia

ActionAid International, India—Christy Abraham
AIDS Alliance India—Padma Buggineni
HIV + Cambodia—Men Thol
Technical Support Facility—Jemal Ahmed
Vietnamese National Network of PLHIV (VNP+)— Venkatesan Chakrapani, Kiran Dhillon, and Do Dang Dong

Europe

AIDS Orphan—Ian Govendir

Egmont Trust, UK—Linnea Renton

International HIV/AIDS Alliance, UK— Anton Kerr, Sam McPherson, Jayne Obeng,, Mike Podmore, Eduardo Romero, and Jill Russell

London University College—Lorraine Sherr

Save the Children International—Alice Fay

Starfish Charity—Elizabeth West

Strategies for Hope Trust, UK—Glen Williams

Thembisa Development Consulting—Nigel Taylor

UK Consortium on AIDS and International Development—Roger Drew and Ben Simms

Women and Children First, UK—Ruth Duebbert

World Vision International—Stuart Kean

Latin America

Alliance Against AIDS, Belize—Rodel Beltran

International Community of Women Living with HIV/AIDS in Latin America (ICW Latina)—Arely Cano Meza

Latin American and the Caribbean Council of AIDS Services Organization (LACCASO)—Alessandra Nilo

Middle East and North Africa

Islamic Relief—Mamoun Abuarqub

North America

Center for Global Health Equity, Tulane University School of Public Health and Tropical Medicine—Carl Kendall

Huairou Commission—Shannon Hayes

International Agencies and Foundations

The Bill and Melinda Gates Foundation—Gina Dallabetta and Tisha Wheeler

The Global Fund to Flight AIDS, Tuberculosis and Malaria—Eddy Addai, *Ryuchi Komatsu, Margaret Kugonza, Daniel Low-Beer, and Mick Matthews*

PEPFAR and USAID—Anjabebu Asrat, Paul Bouey, John Novak, Beverly Nyberg, and Llana Salaiz

UNAIDS— Michel Bartos, Edy Beck, Barbara De Zalduondo, Sally Smith, and Kate Thompson

UNICEF—Priscilla Idele and Rachel Yates

Evaluation Approach and Methods

Abstract

Appendix C provides a more detailed description of the evaluation methodology than chapter 2, including the participatory approach that was followed.

Introduction

This appendix describes in detail the approach and methods used in this evaluation. The consultative process is also addressed.

Goal

The overall goal of the evaluation was to examine and report in a rigorous manner the results achieved at the community level, or in other words, the effects of community responses on HIV and AIDS.

Approach and Guiding Principles

The approach to the overall evaluation followed six guiding principles:

- Be selective: not every single aspect of the epidemic and the response can be evaluated.
- Use a phased-in approach.
- Use a mixed-method approach and make the evaluation as rigorous and robust as possible.
- Utilize existing data if they are current and of high quality; collect primary data—quantitative primarily, but also qualitative and financial, and use triangulation.
- Establish partnerships and a consultative process with experienced researchers, civil society, and partners.
- Consult and validate with national authorities and stakeholders.

Evaluation Design

Selective Evaluation

In theory, one would wish to study more aspects of the community response in more countries and regions affected by the HIV epidemic. In practice, this was not possible as the logistical implications would have been overwhelming. Instead the approach used was to (a) select a group of countries that would be sufficiently diverse to present different forms of community responses, (b) evaluate the various dimensions of the community response as a whole in a few countries, and (c) evaluate different interventions in other countries so that in the end a comprehensive package of interventions would have been evaluated. This implied that while the community response as a whole would be evaluated in a limited number of countries, specific interventions or programs would be evaluated in others.

The overall approach is illustrated in figure C.1 as a puzzle. The assumption made was that the evaluation could not examine every single piece of the puzzle. However, it would examine enough of the key pieces to get a sense of the overall figure and see what story it could tell.

Countries were selected on the basis of several criteria that included (a) a track record of implementation of community-based interventions, (b) country interest in the evaluation, (c) type of HIV epidemic (both high and low HIV prevalence), (d) type of community response, and (e) the availability of data and/or feasibility of data collection.

The objectives of each study were chosen so that they would cover some, if not all, aspects of the continuum of interventions from prevention to treatment, care, support, and mitigation. To evaluate various dimensions of the community response, the focus of the country evaluations varied. Two evaluations (Kenya and

Figure C.1 A Puzzle Approach to Evaluation

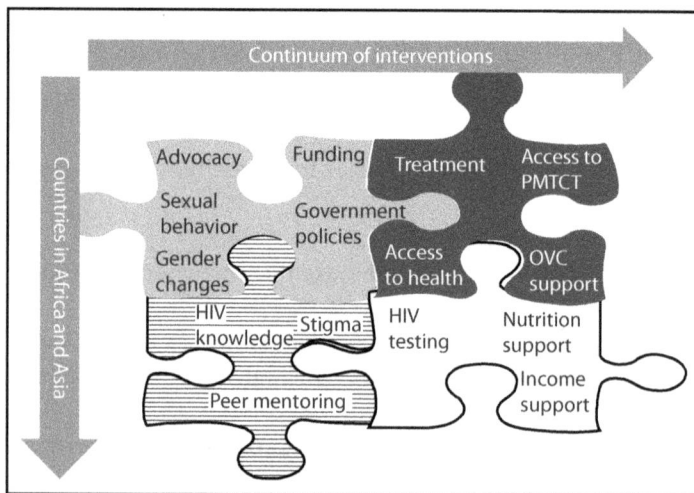

Note: HIV = human immunodeficiency virus, PMTCT = prevention of mother-to-child transmission, OVC = orphans and vulnerable children.

Nigeria) assessed the effects of the intensity (low versus high) of CBO activity at the community level. Another evaluation (Kenya) assessed the effects of home-based testing and counseling. In Burkina Faso, the evaluation examined the effects of prevention programs implemented by CBOs. In Zimbabwe, the protective effects provided by indigenous community group membership (such as burial societies, women groups, sports clubs, and AIDS-related groups) were the focus of the evaluation. The empowerment of groups at high risk of infection and its effects were the subject of two evaluations in India. The effects of peer mentoring on HIV testing and counseling were evaluated in Senegal, while the effects of peer support on adherence and nutritional support for antiretroviral treatment were the focus of the evaluation in South Africa. Finally, the study in Lesotho investigated the socioeconomic determinants of HIV-related stigmatization attitudes.

Phased-in Approach

One of the first activities undertaken was a virtual survey of stakeholders, which was conducted to identify the lenses through which to examine community responses and to inform the design of the evaluation. Other in-depth studies followed (figure C.2). The first one concerned the typology of community responses and helped define the various types of community responses that would be represented in the evaluation. The second study provided information on the funding flows from donors to CSOs and on the activities and resources of small CSOs worldwide (obtained through a survey of more than 100 CBOs), which helped to frame the specific surveys of CBOs that were then carried out in Kenya and Nigeria.

Figure C.2 Design and Implementation of the Evaluation: A Phase-In Approach

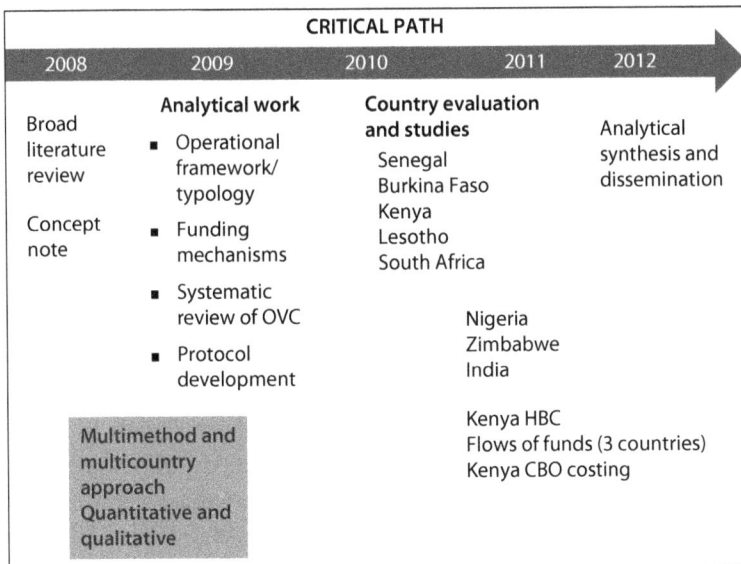

Note: CBO = community-based organization, HBC = home-based care, OVC = orphans and vulnerable children.

The first study in Kenya assessed the effects of CBOs on the continuum of interventions, from prevention to care, support, and mitigation. By covering broad dimensions of the community response, it provided indications of areas where CBOs were having an impact and others where they were not. This evaluation paved the way for the second evaluation of CBO activities in Nigeria. Taken together, these two evaluations indicated the overall effects of community responses, but they also showed that additional studies needed to be carried out in specific areas which were of great interest, such as the effects of home-based counseling and testing, which was assessed in Kenya, and the empowerment effects of high-risk groups, which was studied in India. The evaluations also showed the diversity of CBOs, which prompted a further investigation into the role of indigenous community groups in Zimbabwe.

Mixed-Method Approach

This evaluation applied a mixed-method, multicountry approach to achieve a better understanding of the evaluation results. Quantitative and qualitative analyses, household and CBO surveys, interviews of key informants and local leaders, and desk analyses were carried out. The objective was to generate a comprehensive body of information that would provide robust evidence on the community response (see table C.1). In a mixed-method approach, methods compensate for each other's weaknesses, providing more coherent, reliable, and useful information from which to draw conclusions. The approach is often considered superior to using single methods. Thus, in this mixed-method approach, triangulation becomes a central function to see how data sets confirm, challenge, or explain the findings (World Bank 2012, chapter 11).

Each study design applied research methods most appropriate to the study questions. Three evaluation studies used an experimental design (RCT) with households, individuals, or community randomization. Six studies were quasi-experimental using repeated cross-sectional surveys and propensity score matching or other matching methods to establish comparison groups. Two were analytical studies that used recent Demographic and Health Survey (DHS) data (Lesotho) and data from the evaluation for new in-depth state level analysis (Nigeria). In addition there were two qualitative studies and two-cross cutting studies focusing on OVCs and finance mechanisms. The analytical and desk studies were based on data collected from donors, CBOs, and other survey data.

The experimental and quasi-experimental evaluations used robust methods for establishing a counterfactual within the reality of each specific field setting and limitations of the available data sources. *Experimental designs* are generally viewed as the most rigorous method. By randomly allocating the interventions among beneficiaries, this method creates comparable treatment and provides for control groups that allow causal factors to be identified.[1] This design was applied in Kenya to assess the impact of home-based counseling and testing, in Senegal to evaluate the effects of different sensitization techniques for HIV counseling and testing, and in South Africa to evaluate the impact of peer adherence on antiretroviral treatment.

Table C.1 A Portfolio Approach to Evidence Building

	Experimental design	Quasi-experimental design	CBO funding	Qualitative study	Cross-cutting studies
Evaluation studies					
Burkina Faso		✓			
India		✓ (two)		Component	
Kenya		✓	Component	Component	
Kenya (HBCT)	✓				
Nigeria		✓	Component	Component	
Lesotho					
Senegal	✓				
South Africa	✓				
Zimbabwe		✓	Component	✓	
Analytical, field, and desk studies					
Typology of community response				✓	
Cost structure of CBO budgets in Kenya			✓		
Funding mechanisms					✓
OVC review					✓
Analysis of CBO resources and expenditures in Kenya, Nigeria, Zimbabwe				✓	
Total (15)	3	6	1	3	2

Note: CBO = community-based organization, HBCT = home-based counseling and testing, OVC = orphans and vulnerable children. "Component" means that the qualitative analysis was part of the quantitative household survey.

Quasi-experimental designs were applied in six country studies: Burkina Faso, India (two studies), Kenya (two studies), Nigeria, and Zimbabwe (prospective study). A disadvantage of quasi-experimental methods is that they can confirm an association, but they cannot establish strong statistical causality between an intervention and its effects. However, they offer the major advantage of being able to evaluate wholesale, community-driven programs rather than specific program components.

To overcome the limitations of quasi-experimental studies, the country evaluations were designed so that the same intervention or activities would be evaluated in one or more countries. This allowed the evaluations to reach a somewhat stronger conclusion. When an intervention was found to be associated with a similar outcome in another country, there was a stronger likelihood that the association was not purely coincidental, but could be interpreted as being causal.

Additional information on the community response was provided by qualitative studies and analysis of CBO budgets. In Kenya and Nigeria, the evaluations included four components: (a) a household survey, (b) in-depth interviews with

CBO staff members and key informants from community groups, (c) in-depth interviews with key informants in research communities, and (d) funding alloca- tion data collected from CBOs. In Zimbabwe, two in-depth qualitative analyses of community responses, including the role of grassroots organizations, provided information on the pathways through which behavioral changes were taking place. In India, a background study reported the process by which communities of FSWs and MSM/Ts became empowered. Additional information on the resources mobilized by CBOs came from a three-country analysis of funding flows and resource allocation (India, Kenya, and Nigeria).

Sample sizes: A common limitation of previous analyses of community pro- grams has been their small sample size. To ensure that the results would be as robust as possible, the country evaluations used larger sample sizes (table C.2).

This portfolio of studies allowed for triangulation of data and for the check- ing of the consistency of findings across studies. By providing information on various aspects of the community response, these studies helped identify the results of the community response more broadly and provided some insights into the reasons why these results were achieved. Each single study provides only a partial view of the community response. Taken together, the studies paint a more comprehensive picture of the community response in different contexts.

Evaluation Framework

The design of the evaluation was guided by the causal-logic theory of change shown in figure C.3 as applied to the community response. This figure summa- rizes what is a much more complex pathway linking the community response to

Table C.2   Country Evaluations: Sample Sizes

Countries	Survey sample size
Burkina Faso	44,417 individuals from 8,496 households surveyed in 2007 (National Survey, QUIBB); analysis of prevention at community level
India FSW (Karnataka state)	1,750 (2010 Behavioral Tracking Survey);and 4,700 (two rounds of IBBA in 2005–09); analysis of communities of FSWs
India FSW; MSM (Andhra Pradesh state)	3,557 FSW (2010–11 Behavioral Tracking Survey); 3,546 MSM; analysis of communities of FSWs and MSMs
Kenya	2,715 households; 4,378 individuals in 14 communities (2010 household survey)
Kenya HBCT	3,000 households in 2009–10
Lesotho	14,719 women, 6,114 men (two rounds DHS 2004, 2009)
Nigeria	5,376 households in 28 communities (2011)
Senegal	Data covers 158,178 tests over 15 months from first quarter of 2008 to third quarter of 2009; health districts are randomized in three groups: 9, 19 and 24 for comparison
South Africa	864—four groups of 216 individuals each on ART (2007–11)
Zimbabwe	9,600 women and 6,680 men—four rounds (2,400 women; 1670 men) in 1998–2003; about 200 communities

Note: ART = antiretroviral treatment, DHS = Demographic and Health Survey, FSW = female sex worker, HBCT = home-based counseling and testing, IBBA = Integrated Behavioral and Biological Assessment, MSM = men who have sex with men, QUIBB = Questionnaire on Basic Welfare Indicators.

Figure C.3 The Causal-Logic Theory of Change Linking the Community Response to Improved HIV- and AIDS-Related Results

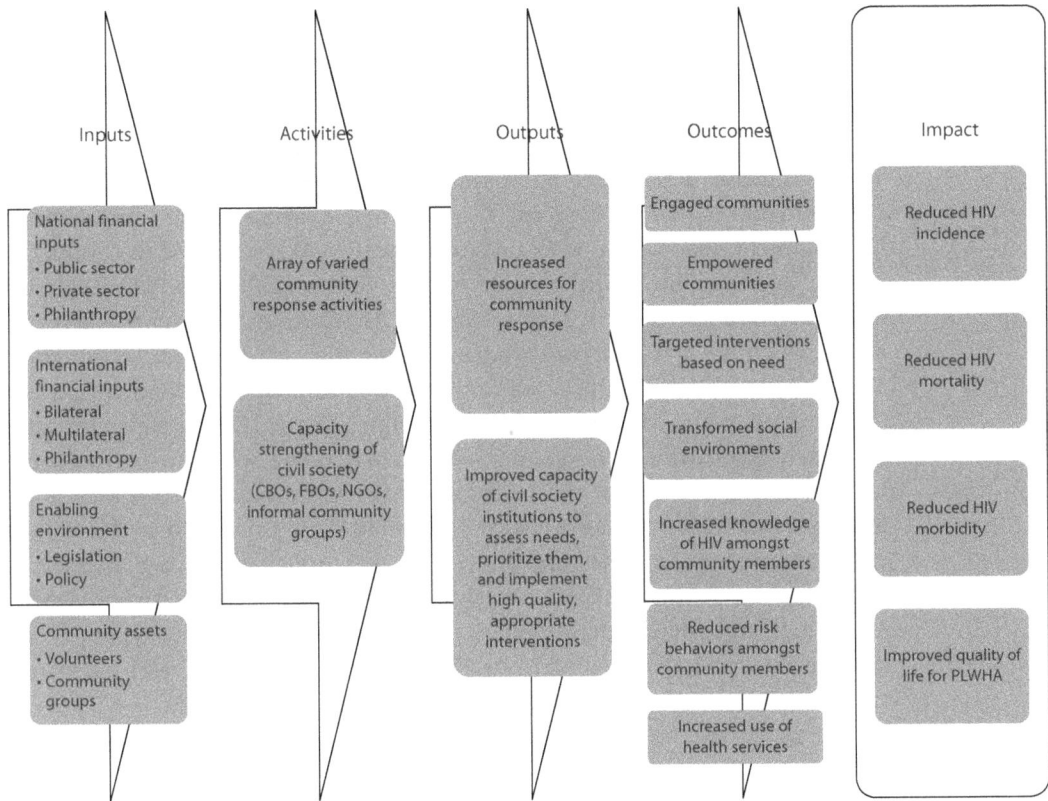

Source: Authors and A. Asrat, USAID Office of HIV/AIDS.
Note: CBO = community-based organization, FBO = faith-based organization, HIV = human immunodeficiency virus, NGO = nongovernmental organization, PLWHA = people living with HIV and AIDS.

HIV outcomes. It is shown here mainly to indicate the assumed relationships from inputs to impacts.

Inputs of the Community Response

The premise of this pathway is that the strength of the community response is affected by the context in which it operates, the resources that community-based groups can mobilize, and the infrastructure and services provided by the government and the private sector. These inputs were analyzed by carrying out a series of studies that provided a typology of community response and that generated information on donor funding for the community response, the resources mobilized by community-based organizations, and their methods for recording expenditures.

Outputs and Outcomes

The hypothesis underlying the theory of change is that differences in the strength of community responses would increase the utilization of HIV and AIDS services, change sexual behaviors, and facilitate social transformation in the form of reduced violence, reduced stigmatization of groups at high risk of infection, and altered gender relations. The final step is the hypothesis that these changes lead to reduced HIV incidence and improved welfare.

Consultative Process

The evaluation design and implementation benefitted from the continuous involvement of two partners. The UK's Department for International Development joined early on as a strategic partner and co-funded the evaluation effort. The UK Consortium on AIDS and International Development joined the evaluation as a civil society partner. The UK Consortium has over 90 members, all of which are networks with organizations that are involved in the global response to HIV and AIDS, as well as broader health and development goals.

The explicit involvement of civil society through the UK Consortium proved extremely worthwhile. The consortium facilitated the work of the evaluation team with other CSOs at the global and national levels, helped ensure active involvement of CSOs in the design and planning of the evaluation, and facilitated the sharing of findings virtually and in person—bringing together a variety of CSOs, representatives of CSO networks, researchers, specialists, national AIDS authorities, and donor representatives. These efforts, sustained throughout the 3 years of the evaluation, helped to strengthen the design and focus of the evaluations and create a platform for the validation and use of findings.

Dialogues with national AIDS authorities and stakeholders took place at an early stage to determine whether the evaluation should take place, and, if so, how best to implement it. These discussions helped shape the country evaluation approach, identify teams, and facilitate the active participation of National AIDS Commission's staff in the evaluation. Consultations were also held at the local level within countries.

Limitations

The evaluation approach and methodology helped answer the questions that were raised at the outset. However, a number of limitations need to be noted:

- The evaluation of the *community response defined as a geographic location* does not make it possible to link specific interventions with specific results, as many actors are involved in the community response.
- The evaluation provides results that may not be transferable to all countries without additional analysis of community characteristics and the overall environment (for example, laws, government role, and so on).
- The evaluation does not indicate whether the community response is cost-effective. To answer that question, country-specific analyses would have to be carried out.

Note

1. Random allocation ensures that no systematic differences between intervention groups in factors, known and unknown, may affect the outcome. Other study designs, including quasi-experimental studies, can detect associations between an intervention and an outcome, but they cannot rule out the possibility that the association was caused by a third factor linked to both interventions.

Bibliography

Burkina Faso Evaluation Report. 2011. Social and Individual Behaviour Change Initiated by Prevention Activities and Antiretroviral Treatment Provision in Burkina Faso. Washington, DC: World Bank.*

India Evaluation Report. 2011. Evaluation of Community Mobilization and Empowerment in Relation to HIV Prevention among Female Sex Workers in Karnataka State, South India. Washington, DC: World Bank.*

———. 2012a. Using Data to Understand Programmatic Shifts in the Avahan HIV Prevention Program at the Community Level. Washington, DC: World Bank.*

———. 2012b. Community Collectivization and Its Association with Selected Outcomes among Female Sex Workers and High-Risk Men Who Have Sex with Men/Transgenders in Andhra Pradesh, India. Washington, DC: World Bank.*

Kenya Evaluation Report. 2011. Effects of the Community Response on HIV and AIDS in Kenya. Washington, DC: World Bank.*

Kenya HBCT Evaluation Report. 2012. The Links between Home-Based HIV Counseling and Testing and HIV Stigma in Western Kenya. Washington, DC: World Bank.*

Lesotho Evaluation Report. 2011. Combating the AIDS Pandemic in Lesotho by Understanding Beliefs and Behaviors. Washington, DC: World Bank.*

Nigeria Evaluation Report 2011. Effects of the Community Response to HIV and AIDS in Nigeria. Washington, DC: World Bank.*

Senegal Evaluation Report. 2010. HIV/AIDS Sensitization, Social Mobilization and Peer-Mentoring: Evidence from a Randomized Experiment. Washington, DC: World Bank.*

South Africa Evaluation Report. 2011. Timely Peer Adherence and Nutritional Support in Free State Province's Public Sector Antiretroviral Treatment Program. Washington, DC: World Bank.*

World Bank. 2012. Building Better Policies: The Nuts and Bolts of Monitoring and Evaluation Systems. G. Lopez-Acevedo, P. Krause, and K. MacKay, eds. Washington, DC: World Bank.

Zimbabwe Evaluation Report. 2011a. Social Capital and AIDS Competent Communities: Evidence from Eastern Zimbabwe. Washington, DC: World Bank.*

———. 2011b. Evaluation of Community Response to HIV and AIDS: Building Competent Communities: Evidence from Eastern Zimbabwe. Washington, DC: World Bank.*

———. 2012. Similarities and Differences in the Community Response to HIV and AIDS in Matabeleland South and Manicaland. Washington, DC: World Bank.*

*See names of contributors to this report in appendix A.

Design and Methods of Country Evaluations

Abstract

Appendix D offers a compact summary of the studies that were carried out.

Summary

BURKINA FASO: *Social and Individual Behavior Change Initiated by HIV/AIDS Prevention Activities in Burkina Faso* (Burkina Faso Evaluation Report 2011).

Program Implementer	Village committees to fight HIV/AIDS. HIV-related services delivered locally by NGOs and associations.
Interventions	Individual participation at least once in a community-based prevention activity in the past 12 months, that is, HIV prevention activities such as debates, movies, discussions with peer educators, theater plays, and other activities.
Population Groups	General population 15 years old and above. 44,417 individuals from 8,496 households surveyed in 2007 (national survey, Questionnaire on Basic Welfare Indicators, or QUIBB).
Evaluation Design and Methods	Quasi-experimental study with matching of communities:
	Data were collected using the Questionnaire Unifié des Indicateurs du Bien-être au Burkina Faso (QUIBB), a nationally representative household survey on living conditions (education, income, and health—including HIV/AIDS and sexual practices) in 2008, 2009, and 2010. A two-stage random sample was used that was representative of the country's 13 regions and 425 enumeration areas.
	Sample size: $n = 44{,}417$ individuals, 15 years old and above in 8,496 households.
	First, the study ran probit regressions of the various behavior variables with enumeration area fixed effects. It revealed a potential self-selection of individuals: individuals more susceptible to participate in prevention activities could be the ones with riskier behaviors. To address this bias, the evaluation studied the effect of a variable unlikely to be affected by individual decisions, namely the location of the respondent in a province where the World Bank Multi-Country HIV/AIDS Program (MAP) aimed at implementing community-based programs, which has been operating since 2002.
RESULTS	
Knowledge	Small and mixed effects on knowledge with effects varying by gender.
Access to and Utilization of HIV-Related Services	Use of HIV testing services in the past 12 months: no significant effect.
Risk Behavior	• Condom use with first partner: significant positive effect for women ($p < .10$).
	• Condom use with second partner: significant positive effect for men ($p < .01$).
	• No significant effect on HIV-related knowledge, abstinence, and fidelity.
Social Transformation	• Personal expression of stigmatization: no significant effect.
	• Personal belief that the community stigmatizes infected persons: significant positive effect for men and women ($p < .05$).

INDIA: *Evaluation of Community Mobilization and Empowerment in Relation to HIV Prevention among Female Sex Workers in Karnataka State, South India* (India Evaluation Report 2011).

Program Implementer	The program was delivered by the Karnataka Health Promotion Trust (KHPT), which is a partnership between the University of Manitoba (Canada) and the Karnataka State AIDS Prevention Society (KSAPS) and is part of the larger Avahan program.
Interventions	• Community collectivization for behavioral change and building an enabling environment. • Clinical services for STIs and counseling managed by the community. • Local advocacy including police sensitization, crisis response, and community advisory committees.
Population Groups	1,750 FSWs in 21 districts of Karnataka state (2010 Behavioral Tracking Survey).
Evaluation Design and Methods	Quasi-experimental study using three sources of data: Behavioral Tracking Survey (BTS) (2010): • Random sample of FSW in five districts in 2010 ($n = 350$ FSW per district). • Survey data were used to identify associations with "power within" (self-efficacy), "power with" (collective efficacy), and "power over resources" (collective agency). • Survey data were used to identify associations with individual behavioral outcomes using propensity score matching (PSM) to account for differences in CBO members and nonmembers. Integrated Behavioral and Biological Assessments (IBBA): • Random sample of FSW in five districts in 2006 and 2010 ($n = 400$ FSW per district). • Survey data were used to identify associations with individual biological outcomes using PSM to account for differences in CBOs members and non-members. Qualitative study: • Narrative case studies were conducted.
RESULTS	
Access to and Utilization of HIV-Related Services	For all districts, "power within" was associated with the number of visits to health clinics during the last 6 months ($p < .05$).
Risk Behavior	"Power with" was associated with increased condom use with occasional and regular clients (after adjustment, statistically significantly $p < .05$).
Social Transformation	After adjustment, the following associations were statistically significantly ($p < .05$): • All three domains of empowerment: "power within," "power with," and "power over" were associated with intensity of program delivery at the district level. • "Power with" and "power within" were associated with self-efficacy for service utilization. • "Power within" was associated with self-efficacy for condom use with nonpaying regular partners. • "Power with" was associated with self-efficacy for condom use with clients. • In the high intensity areas, "power with" was associated with more autonomy and less experience of violence. After adjustment and using PSM, membership of a CBO was associated with: • Reduced experience of violence ($p < .001$); • Reduced police coercion ($p < .001$); and, • Increased ownership of identity card ($p < .05$).
HIV Incidence and Health Status	Being a member of a CBO among matched FSWs was associated with: • Reduced STI (chlamydia and gonorrhea) ($p < .001$) • Reduced active syphilis ($p < .05$) • Reduced HIV prevalence (but not significant).

Note: "Power within" was created from variables that measured the degree to which the respondent did not feel ashamed to be identified as an FSW, and had confidence to seek advice and give their opinion in public. "Power with" was created from variables that measured the respondent's confidence in the ability of sex workers to band together for various purposes, whether they could rely on other sex workers for support, whether they had a network of peers they could trust, and whether they were members of community groups and participated in public events.

INDIA (Andhra Pradesh State): *Community Collectivization and Its Association with Selected Outcomes among Female Sex Workers and High-Risk Men Who Have Sex with Men/Transgenders in Andhra Pradesh, India* (India Evaluation Report 2012b).

Program Implementer	Avahan program. The program was implemented by the Hindustan Latex Family Planning Promotion Trust (HLFPPT) and the India AIDS Alliance, Andhra Pradesh.
Interventions	• Community mobilization of high-risk groups • Building an enabling environment • Community crisis response • Engagement on issues of rights, entitlements, and stigma reduction
Population Groups	3,557 FSWs (2010–11 Behavioral Tracking Survey) 3,546 high-risk men who have sex with men/trans-genders (MSM/T).
Evaluation Design and Methods	Behavioral Tracking Survey (BTS) in 2010/11 among FSWs and MSM/T: • Survey interviews were conducted with a stratified random sample of community groups. • Data were collected using a cross-sectional survey in sites with the Avahan program using conventional cluster sampling and time-location cluster sampling. • Sample size: n = 3,557 FSWs from nine districts; n = 2,399 HR-MSM from six districts.

RESULTS FOR FSWs

Access to and Utilization of HIV-Related Services	FSWs: STI treatment from government referral health facilities: Collectivization: Proportion of FSWs visiting a government health facility for STI treatment was significantly higher among those with medium versus low collectivization (60.4 versus 42.2 percent, aOR: 2.1, 95 percent CI: 1.3–3.2). The same is true for two measures of collectivization: collective efficacy and collective agency. Collective action: proportion of FSWs who reported visiting government health facilities for STI treatment among those reporting a high degree of collective action was lower (44.3 percent) compared with that (59.1 percent) among FSWs with low collective action (aOR: 0.5, 95 percent CI: 0.3–0.8).
Risk Behavior	Collectivization: Consistent condom use with occasional clients increased significantly with increases in the degree of collectivization from low to high (74.5 versus 83.8 percent, aOR: 1.8, 95 percent CI: 1.2–2.6). Collectivization: Consistent condom use with regular clients also increased from 66.4 percent among those reporting a low degree of collectivization to 75.9 percent among those reporting a high degree of collectivization (aOR: 1.7, 95 percent CI: 1.2–2.4). The same result holds for two measures of collectivization: collective efficacy and collective action.
Social Transformation	FSWs who reported a high degree of collectivization compared to those who reported a low level of collectivization were about three times more likely to have high self-efficacy for condom use with clients (82.1 versus 65.0 percent, aOR: 2.5, 95 percent CI: 1.6–3.7). Self-efficacy: The proportion of FSWs who reported high self-efficacy for service utilization from government health facilities was significantly higher among those reporting a medium or high degree of collectivization than among those with a low level of collectivization (low: 38.9 percent; medium: 56.2 percent, aOR: 2.0, 95 percent CI: 1.6–2.5; high: 78.4 percent, aOR: 5.5, 95 percent CI: 3.9–7.8). Self-confidence: the proportion of FSWs with high self-confidence in expressing opinions was lower among FSWs with a low level of collectivization (35.1 percent) compared to those with a medium level of collectivization (54.5 percent, aOR: 2.3, 95 percent CI: 1.8–2.8) or a high level of collectivization (75.8 percent, aOR: 5.9, 95 percent CI: 4.1–8.4).

RESULTS FOR MSM/T

Access to and Utilization of HIV-Related Services	For MSM/T: The results did not reveal any association of visiting government health facilities for STI treatment with either participation in public events or collective efficacy.

table continues next page

INDIA: *Using Data to Understand Programmatic Shifts in the Avahan HIV Prevention Program at the Community Level* (India Evaluation Report 2012a).

Program Implementer	Avahan program.
Interventions	Community group mobilization measured by Community Ownership and Preparedness tool. Participatory planning with NGOs and community groups.
Evaluation Design and Methods	Survey of nine community groups for FSWs and HR-MSM in 2008–10, and 2009/10.
RESULTS	• Higher participation of the community in all aspects of program: "program implementation," "program management," "program monitoring," and "policy decisions." • Reductions in violence by police. • Community response to crisis undertaken with no program involvement. • CBOs aware of laws relating to their rights and assumed primary role in negotiating for rights on behalf of communities (those at greatest risk of HIV; high-risk groups). • CBOs are working with other civil society organizations (women's organizations, politicians, advocates, and the media).

INDIA (Andhra Pradesh State): *Community Collectivization and Its Association with Selected Outcomes among Female Sex Workers and High-Risk Men Who Have Sex with Men/Transgenders in Andhra Pradesh, India* (India Evaluation Report 2012b). *(continued)*

Risk Behavior	Participation in any public event: HR-MSM who participated in any public event compared to their counterparts were significantly more likely to use a condom consistently with both paid partners (74.3 percent, versus 48.1 percent, aOR: 3.3, 95 percent CI: 2.1–5.2) and nonpaying partners (75.3 percent, versus 54.9 percent, aOR: 2.7, 95 percent CI: 2.0–3.6).
	Collective efficacy: A higher proportion of HR-MSM who reported high collective efficacy used condoms consistently with paying partners (76.5 percent) compared with the proportion (64.0 percent) among those reporting a low level of collective efficacy (aOR: 1.9, 95 percent CI: 1.5–2.3).
	No significant difference could be observed in the consistent condom use with paid partners between those who reported high collective efficacy and those who did not.
Social Transformation	Self-efficacy: MSM/Ts who participated in any public event compared to their counterparts were significantly more likely to have high self-efficacy for condom use (74.4 versus 63.4 percent, aOR:1.8, 95 percent CI: 1.5–2.3); high self-efficacy for service utilization from government health facilities (59.5 versus 38.0 percent, aOR:2.5, 95 percent CI: 2.0–3.1); and high self-confidence in expressing opinions (60.7 versus 50.9 percent, aOR:1.5, 95 percent CI: 1.2–1.8).
	MSM/Ts who reported high collective efficacy compared with their counterparts were significantly more likely to have high self-efficacy for condom use (84.7 versus 51.6 percent, aOR: 4.9, 95 percent CI: 4.1–6.0); high self-efficacy for service utilization from government health facilities (66.9 versus 35.8 percent, aOR: 3.6, 95 percent CI: 3.0–4.3); and high self-confidence in expressing opinions (70.8 versus 39.0 percent, aOR: 3.7, 95 percent CI: 3.1–4.4).

Note: "Collective efficacy" is the belief of the affected community in its power to work together to effect change. "Collective agency" is the choice, control, and power that poor or marginalized groups have to act for themselves to claim their rights (whether civil, political, economic, social, or cultural) and to hold others accountable for these rights. "Collective action" is the strategic and organized activities by mobilized community members to increase the community's visibility in wider society and present or enact its agenda for change (for example, through rallies, demonstrations, or meetings with stakeholders).

KENYA: *Effects of the Community Response to HIV and AIDS in Kenya* (Kenya Evaluation Report 2011).

Program Implementer	This was not an evaluation of a specific intervention but an assessment of the impact of a strong community response, operationalized as a high level of CBO engagement on HIV- and AIDS-related outcomes. In Kenya, CBO engagement was measured by the proportion of respondents who were aware of HIV-related services provided by CBOs in their community.
Interventions	Research questions were the following: Do communities with a stronger community-based response show significant differences in: • Health outcomes compared to communities with a weaker response? • Access to and utilization of HIV and AIDS services compared to communities with a weaker response? • Knowledge, attitudes, perception, and behavior compared to communities with a weaker response? • Social transformation indicators compared to communities with a weaker response? *and* • What are the funding sources of CBO budgets and how is this funding used to support community-based activities for prevention, treatment, care, and mitigation?
Population Groups	Kenya: 3,000 households in 2009/10.
Evaluation Design and Methods	Quasi-experimental study with matching: • The study involved 14 matched pairs of communities with a high community response (study group) and a low community response (comparison group); there was some post-hoc reassignment to the groups based on CBO awareness in the respective communities. • Data were collected using a household survey in 2010 ($n = 4,378$ individuals). Qualitative study: • CBOs and key informant interviews were conducted ($n = 25$ CBOs and 58 individuals).
RESULTS	
Access to and Utilization of HIV-Related Services	No statistically significant association between CBO engagement and awareness, and reported availability and reported use of HIV/AIDS-related services.
Risk Behavior	• Respondents in the study communities had higher odds of knowing that (a) having one, uninfected partner reduces chances of HIV transmission (OR: 9.26, 95 percent CI: 3.09–27.7); (b) using a condom reduces the chances of becoming infected with HIV (OR: 14.67, 95 percent CI: 7.73–27.85); and (c) the chances of vertical transmission of HIV can be reduced by PMTCT prophylaxis (ORP: 3.48, 95 percent CI: 1.92–7.70). • Respondents in the study communities had higher odds than respondents in the comparison communities of reporting consistent condom use with all sex partners in the last 12 months (OR: 4.09, 95 percent CI: 2.30–7.27).
Social Transformation	• Respondents in the study communities were about 25 percent more likely to be aware of institutions that promote and protect children's rights (OR: 1.25, 95 percent CI: 1.62–7.46). • Significant association with indicators of institutional social capital: households in the study group reported about two more people than households in the comparison group who voted in national elections (β: 1.85, SE: 0.56) and in local elections (β: 1.7, SE: 0.86), and 1.3 persons more who participated in electoral campaigns (β: 1.28, SE: 0.33). • No statistically significant associations between CBO engagement and cognitive social capital and gender norms. Key informants did not observe any direct impact of CBOs on social capital and gender norms. Instead, increased awareness of political rights and the value of getting together to solve community problems were credited to changes in values and increasing awareness of social and political rights. • Increases in female enrolment in education and perceived declines in violence against women were attributed to changes in national policies: the introduction of free primary-level education and the adoption of legislation protecting women from violence. • Declining levels of stigma were linked to value changes and increased awareness and knowledge of AIDS at the community level, which, on the basis of the interview data, cannot be directly attributed to CBO activities.

KENYA: (Home-Based Counseling and Testing): *The Links between Home-Based HIV Counseling and Testing, and HIV/AIDS Stigma in Western Kenya* (Kenya HBCT Evaluation Report 2012).

Program Implementer	The Academic Model Providing Access to Healthcare (AMPATH), a healthcare collaboration in Western Kenya, provided home-based HIV counseling and testing (HBCT) to all community members. Community leaders mobilized community members through road shows and town hall meetings to encourage HBCT uptake in advance of the testing event.
Interventions	• Community leaders were educated about HIV/AIDS and the HBCT program and timeline. • Facilitators, usually drawn from the local community, worked with local government to explain the HBCT program to the community. • Locally based counselors visited all households in the community to provide voluntary counseling and testing to all adults in the household. HIV-tests and associated counseling were administered within the household and couples were encouraged to test together. • Individuals who tested positive for HIV were referred to the local AMPATH treatment facility.
Population Groups	• Community leaders: political, social, and religious leaders. • Community members: all adult members of the target communities were offered home-based counseling and testing; ~70 percent participated. • Sample size: 3,000 households in 2009/10.
RESULTS	Randomized controlled trial: • Geographical locations were randomized to a study group receiving home-based counseling and testing (HBCT) and a non-intervention control group receiving HBCT at a later date. • Data were collected using a household survey in 2009 and 2011 (n = ~3,300 individuals).
Risk Behavior	• HIV knowledge and reported condom use not affected strongly or consistently.
Social Transformation	• Decreased stigmatization attitudes among community leaders ($p < .05$). • Unclear effect on community member's stigmatization attitudes.

Lesotho: *Combating the AIDS Pandemic in Lesotho by Understanding Beliefs and Behaviors towards Stigmatization* (Lesotho Evaluation Report 2011).

Program	This was not an evaluation of a specific intervention, but rather a descriptive analysis of the characteristics of adults who have stigmatization attitudes toward PLHIV.
Population Groups	14,719 women, 6,114 men (two rounds DHS 2004, 2009).
Evaluation Design and Methods	Descriptive study: Data from the 2004 and 2009 rounds of the Lesotho Demographic and Health Survey (LDHS) were analyzed using five questions measuring respondents' attitudes towards PLHIV (representative sample of 14,719 women and 6,114 men of reproductive age (15–49 years). Respondents were living in households in the 10 districts of Lesotho, and the survey included both urban and rural areas. Among the individuals eligible to be interviewed, a random sample of 12,178 individuals (6,869 women; 5,309 men) was selected and tested for HIV. Data analysis focused on (a) the percentages of women and men who express stigmatization attitudes toward PLHIV by background characteristics and (b) the extent to which specific socioeconomic factors (age, education, location, wealth, and traditional circumcision) contribute to HIV stigmatization attitudes in women and men.
RESULTS	
Access to and Utilization of HIV-Related Services	HIV/AIDS stigmatization attitudes are negatively associated with the probability of HIV testing and of obtaining HIV test results ($p < .01$).
Social Transformation	HIV/AIDS stigmatization attitudes are negatively associated with education, wealth, and urban status, and positively associated with Catholic religion for women and traditional circumcision for men ($p < .01$).

NIGERIA: *Effects of the Community Response to HIV and AIDS in Nigeria* (Nigeria Evaluation Report 2011).

Program Implementer	This was not an evaluation of a specific intervention, but rather an assessment of the impact of a strong community response, operationalized as a high level of CBO engagement in HIV- and AIDS-related outcomes. CBO engagement was measured by the number of CBOs per 100,000 present in communities.
Interventions	Research questions included: Do communities with a stronger community-based response show significant differences in: • Health outcomes compared to communities with a weaker response? • Access to and utilization of HIV and AIDS services compared to communities with a weaker response? • Knowledge, attitudes, perception, and behavior compared to communities with a weaker response? • Social transformation indicators compared to communities with a weaker response? *And* • What are the funding sources of CBOs' budgets and how is this funding used to support community-based activities for prevention, treatment, care, and mitigation?
Population Groups	Nigeria: 5,376 households in 28 communities (2011).
Evaluation Design and Methods	Quasi-experimental study with matching community pairs: The study involved 28 matched pairs of communities with a high community response (study group) and a low community response (comparison group). There was some post-hoc reassignment to the groups based on CBO awareness in the respective communities. Data were collected using a household survey in 2010 and 2011 ($n = 5,376$ individuals) Qualitative study: CBO and key informant interviews were conducted ($n = 45$ CBOs and 65 individuals).
RESULTS	
Access to and Utilization of HIV-Related Services	Statistically significant associations between CBO engagement and reported use of (a) any HIV/AIDS-related services (aOR: 2.06; 95 percent CI: 1.21–3.50); (b) prevention services (aOR: 4.39; 95 percent CI: 1.56–12.35); and (c) care and support services (aOR: 2.49; 95 percent CI: 1.16–5.33). No statistically significant associations between CBO engagement and HIV testing.
Risk Behavior	No statistically significant associations between CBO engagement and AIDS-related knowledge and sexual risk behaviors.
Social Transformation	No statistically significant associations between CBO engagement and AIDS-related stigmatization. No statistically significant association between CBO engagement and cognitive social capital. Interviews with key informants suggest that other factors (poverty, crime, national policies, and increasing educational attainment) rather than CBO engagement had affected social capital in the evaluation communities.

SENEGAL: *HIV/AIDS Sensitization, Social Mobilization and Peer-Mentoring: Evidence from a Randomized Experiment* (Senegal Evaluation Report 2010).

Program Implementer	CBOs (either funded or unfunded for intervention delivery).
Interventions	• Standard social sensitization activities (unfunded) including education about HIV/AIDS and voluntary HIV counseling and testing (HCT). • Social sensitization activities (funded). • Peer education about HIV/AIDS and HCT and peer mentoring.
Population Groups	Adults: data cover 158,178 tests over 15 months from first quarter of 2008 to third quarter of 2009.

table continues next page

SENEGAL: *HIV/AIDS Sensitization, Social Mobilization and Peer-Mentoring: Evidence from a Randomized Experiment* (Senegal Evaluation Report 2010). *(continued)*

Evaluation Design and Methods	Randomized controlled trial:
	Health districts were randomized to two study groups receiving either funding or sensitization ($n = 9$ districts) or receiving funding and peer mentoring ($n = 19$ districts) and one comparison group receiving no funding and providing sensitization ($n = 24$ districts).
	Data from routinely collected administrative sources in the health districts were used.
RESULTS	
Access to and Utilization of HIV-Related Services	Peer mentoring by CBOs increased by 90 percent the number of individuals who attend pre-test counseling and get tested, and doubles the number of individuals who picked up their test results.
	Funded standard sensitization techniques appear ineffective.
	For HIV-positive individuals, both approaches increased the number of individuals who attend post-test counseling and the number of their partners being tested.

SOUTH AFRICA: *Timely Peer Adherence and Nutritional Support in Free State Province's Public Sector Antiretroviral Treatment Program* (South Africa Evaluation Report 2011).

Program Implementer	Trained peer adherence supporters from the communities who conducted twice-weekly visits to ART patients.
Interventions	• Treatment and support provided in the existing program.
	• Bi-weekly visits by trained antiretroviral (ARV) peer adherence supporter.
	• Nutritional supplement (canned food).
Population Groups	Adults (18+ years) who initiated ART in the past 4 weeks and reside in a community with a phase- I ART clinic in Free State province.
	Four groups of 216 households (2007–11).
Evaluation Design and Methods	Randomized controlled trial:
	Patients and their households were randomized to 3 study groups: Group A receiving either ART ($n = 216$) and the standard support provided by the clinic; Group B receiving the same intervention ($n = 216$) as Group A plus twice weekly visits from a peer adherence supporter; or Group C receiving the same intervention ($n = 216$) as Group B plus a nutritional supplement (that is, two cans of food) and, one non-intervention comparison group ($n = 208$).
	Fifty peer adherence supporters were recruited at each site and assigned each eight participants.
	Data were collected using a patient survey, patient clinical records, a household survey, and a facility survey.
RESULTS	
Access to and Utilization of HIV-Related Services	Delays in scheduled clinic visits for study participants visited twice-weekly by a peer adherence supporter were statistically significantly lower than for study participants not receiving any peer adherence support (-15.8 days; $p < .05$; 95 percent CI -29.1 to -2.4).
	For visits to the clinic, nutritional support offers no additional benefit above community peer adherence.
	Delays in scheduled hospital visits were statistically significantly lower only for study participants receiving both adherence and nutritional support (-32.5 days; $p < .01$; 95 percent CI -56.7 to -8.4).

ZIMBABWE: *Evaluations of Community Response to HIV and AIDS. Building Competent Communities: Evidence from Eastern Zimbabwe* (Zimbabwe Evaluation Report 2011).

Program Implementer	This was not an evaluation of a specific intervention, but rather an assessment of the spontaneous response from indigenous local community groups including: rotating credit societies, burial societies, women's groups, youth groups, farmers' groups, cooperatives, sports clubs, political parties, church groups, and AIDS-related groups. Case study of community response to peer education (1998–2003). Case study of cash transfer programs (randomized controlled trials) in 2009–11.
Interventions	Participation in community groups at baseline and follow-up. Community groups and effects on villages.
Population Groups	Adult population Four rounds: 2,374 women and 1,673 men in 1998–2003 (HIV incidence analysis); 3,446 women and 1,812 men in 2003–08 (service use analysis); 200 communities (villages).
Evaluation Design and Methods	Prospective cohort study: • Four rounds (1998–2008) of data from a prospective population-based open cohort survey (Manicaland Study) were used including four strata: small towns (2), estates (4), roadside (2), and subsistence farming (4). • Prospective analysis of the cohort data was conducted controlling for prior risk behavior and other characteristics (individual and community-level effects). • Sample size: Four rounds; 2,374 women and 1,673 men in 1998–2003 (HIV incidence analysis); 3,446 women and 1,812 men in 2003–08 (service use analysis); 200 communities (villages). Qualitative study: • Focus group discussions, key informant interviews, and direct observations.
RESULTS	
Access to and Utilization of HIV-Related Services	• Women participating in community activities were quicker to take up new HIV services such as voluntary counseling and testing for HIV infection and prevention of mother-to-child transmission services ($p < .01$). • Women living in villages with greater female community participation had faster uptake of services ($p < .01$). Fewer positive effects were seen for men. • In a few instances, community participation had a negative effect on the development of HIV competence.
Risk Behavior	For women, participation in community groups (and particularly in multiple groups) was associated with a faster adoption of lower-risk sexual behaviors ($p < .01$).
Social Transformation	Individuals who participated in community groups were less likely to have maintained or acquired stigmatization attitudes towards people living with AIDS ($p < .05$).
HIV Incidence	For women, participation in community groups (and particularly in multiple groups) was associated with reduced HIV incidence ($p < .01$). Women living in villages with greater female community participation was associated with lower HIV-infection rates ($p < .01$).

Note: CBO = community-based organization, FSW = female sex workers, IEC = information, education, communication, NGO = nongovernmental organization, PLWHA = people living with HIV and AIDS, STI = sexually transmitted infection, OVC = orphans and vulnerable children.

References

Burkina Faso Evaluation Report. 2011. *Social and Individual Behaviour Change Initiated by Prevention Activities and Antiretroviral Treatment Provision in Burkina Faso.* Washington, DC: World Bank.*

India Evaluation Report. 2011. *Evaluation of Community Mobilization and Empowerment in Relation to HIV Prevention among Female Sex Workers in Karnataka State, South India.* Washington, DC: World Bank.*

————. 2012a. *Using Data to Understand Programmatic Shifts in the Avahan HIV Prevention Program at the Community Level.* Washington, DC: World Bank.*

————. 2012b. *Community Collectivization and Its Association with Selected Outcomes among Female Sex Workes and High-Risk Men Who Have Sex with Men/Transgenders in Andhra Pradesh, India.* Washington, DC: World Bank.*

Kenya Evaluation Report. 2011. *Effects of the Community Response on HIV and AIDS in Kenya.* Washington, DC: World Bank.*

Kenya HBCT Evaluation Report. 2012. *The Links between Home-Based HIV Counseling and Testing and HIV Stigma in Western Kenya.* Washington, DC: World Bank.*

Lesotho Evaluation Report. 2011. *Combating the AIDS Pandemic in Lesotho by Understanding Beliefs and Behaviors.* Washington, DC: World Bank.*

Nigeria Evaluation Report 2011. *Effects of the Community Response to HIV and AIDS in Nigeria.* Washington, DC: World Bank.*

Senegal Evaluation Report. 2010. *HIV/AIDS Sensitization, Social Mobilization and Peer-Mentoring: Evidence from a Randomized Experiment.* Washington, DC: World Bank.*

South Africa Evaluation Report. 2011. *Timely Peer Adherence and Nutritional Support in Free State Province's Public Sector Antiretroviral Treatment Program.* Washington, DC: World Bank.*

Zimbabwe Evaluation Report. 2011. *Evaluation of Community Response to HIV and AIDS: Building Competent Communities: Evidence from Eastern Zimbabwe.* Washington, DC: World Bank.*

---

*See names of contributors to this report in appendix A.

Environmental Benefits Statement

The World Bank is committed to reducing its environmental footprint. In support of this commitment, the Office of the Publisher leverages electronic publishing options and print-on-demand technology, which is located in regional hubs worldwide. Together, these initiatives enable print runs to be lowered and shipping distances decreased, resulting in reduced paper consumption, chemical use, greenhouse gas emissions, and waste.

The Office of the Publisher follows the recommended standards for paper use set by the Green Press Initiative. Whenever possible, books are printed on 50% to 100% postconsumer recycled paper, and at least 50% of the fiber in our book paper is either unbleached or bleached using Totally Chlorine free (TCF), Processed Chlorine Free (PCF), or Enhanced Elemental Chlorine Free (EECF) processes.

More information about the Bank's environmental philosophy can be found at http://crinfo.worldbank.org/crinfo/environmental_responsibility/index.html.

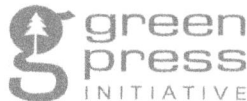

green
press
INITIATIVE

www.ingramcontent.com/pod-product-compliance
Lightning Source LLC
Chambersburg PA
CBHW080616270326
41928CB00016B/3088